NETT

D0233368

THE LEAD SCANDAL ●
THE FIGHT TO SAVE CHILDREN FROM DAMAGE BY LEAD IN PETROL

Des Wilson

As Chairman of CLEAR, the Campaign for Lead-free Air, Des Wilson has for the past two years led the fight to have lead banned from petrol in Britain and the rest of Europe.

In this book he describes the health hazard to children from low-level lead exposure, how in the United States industrialists fought to achieve higher company profits at the expense of public health, and how in Britain politicians, civil servants, and industrialists have combined to keep lead in petrol in the face of widespread parental concern.

Des Wilson is one of Britain's most experienced and best-known campaigners on social issues. He was the first Director of Shelter, National Campaign for the Homeless (1966–71), and is now a member of its Board. He is also Chairman of Friends of the Earth in Britain and is a former National Executive member of the Child Poverty Action Group and the National Council for Civil Liberties.

He is a former Liberal Party parliamentary candidate and a former member of the Party's Council.

As a journalist he has written a weekly column for *The Guardian* (1968–71) and *The Observer* (1971–75), and has contributed over the past 15 years to many other newspapers and magazines, notably *The Times, The London Evening Standard, The New Statesman,* and *The Illustrated London News,* for whom he has been a contributor for ten years and was Deputy Editor from 1979–81. He was Editor of *Social Work Today,* Britain's leading social services magazine (1976–79).

His home is in Bewdley, Worcestershire.

THE LEAD SCANDAL

THE FIGHT TO SAVE
CHILDREN FROM DAMAGE BY LEAD IN PETROL

DES WILSON

Heinemann Educational Books

Heinemann Educational Books Ltd
22 Bedford Square
London WC1B 3HH

LONDON   EDINBURGH   MELBOURNE   AUCKLAND
HONG KONG   SINGAPORE   KUALA LUMPUR   NEW DELHI
IBADAN   NAIROBI   JOHANNESBURG
EXETER (NH)   KINGSTON   PORT OF SPAIN

British Library Cataloguing in Publication Data

Wilson, Des
    The lead scandal.
    1. Children—Care and hygiene   2. Pollution—Great Britain—
    Physiological effect   3. Lead—Environmental aspects
    4. Lead-poisoning—Great Britain
    I. Title
    363.7'384   RA1231.L4

    ISBN 0-435-83945-4
    ISBN 0-435-83946-2 Pbk

Typeset and printed in Great Britain by
Biddles Ltd, Guildford, Surrey

Contents

Acknowledgements

I AM grateful to my colleagues in the CLEAR campaign, Robin Russell Jones and Bob Stephens, for their contribution not only to this book but to the work of CLEAR, for the loyal and generous support they have given me, and for the inspiration I have drawn from their idealism and indefatigable efforts in the cause of child health. When the battle is won, every generation thereafter will be in their debt.

That last sentence also applies to Godfrey Bradman, who has done much more than contribute financially to CLEAR; he has been a loyal supporter and wise adviser and a source of strength to me in many ways.

To these three men I dedicate this book.

I thank, also, Susan Dibb and Patricia Simms with whom I have worked so happily on the CLEAR campaign and without whose support I could not have written the book, and Jane Dunmore, Sam Smith and Tony Smythe for their helpful comments on the manuscript.

Dr. John Jarvis, of John Wiley and Sons, undertook to publish the proceedings of CLEAR's International Symposium. This invaluable scientific publication 'Lead Versus Health: Low Level Lead Exposure and Its Effect on Human Beings', edited by Professor Michael Rutter and Dr. Robin Russell Jones, was due to appear early in 1983. Dr. Jarvis has been understanding of my need to quote extensively from the symposium papers; for that generosity I am most grateful. Readers who wish to delve even deeper into the medical research on this subject will find the Rutter and Russell Jones book most rewarding.

I thank all the authors and publishers whose words are quoted.

Last, but not least, David Hill of Heinemann is the kind of cooperative and helpful publisher everyone hopes to find and few do.

Des Wilson   March 1983

Technical terms

The following abbreviations and measurements appear throughout the book:

Lead in Petrol

g/l — This represents grams per litre of petrol. The British target figure is 0.15 g/l by 1985.

Lead in Blood

ug/dl — This represents micrograms of lead per decilitre (100 millilitres) of blood. The DOE guideline 'safety threshold' in Britain is 25 ug/dl.

Lead Content in Dust, Soil, Food, Paint, etc.

ppm — This represents parts of lead per million parts of dust, soil, food, paint, etc. For instance, the British DOE guideline 'safety level' for lead in dust is 2,000 ppm.

Lead in Air

ug/m^3 — This represents micrograms per cubic metre of air. Britain shares the EEC 'safety level' of 2 ug/m^3.

Abbreviations and Definitions

Pb — Lead.

TEL — Tetraethyl lead – one of the principal additives to petrol.

TML — Tetramethyl lead – the other principal petrol additive.

Anti-knock — Because lead additives reduce engine 'knock', the industries concerned with this practice are often referred to as 'the anti-knock industry'.

Body lead burden — The total amount of lead in a person's body.

LPG — Liquid Petroleum Gas – an alternative to petrol as a fuel for motor vehicles.

MTBE — Methyl tertiary butyl ether – an alternative to lead additives in petrol.

RON — Research octane number, the one normally quoted to specify the grade of petrol being sold.

Organisational abbreviations

EEC — European Economic Community.

WHO — The World Health Organisation.

EPA — The Environmental Protection Agency in the USA.

DOE — Britain's Department of the Environment.

DHSS — Britain's Department of Health and Social Security.

DOT — Britain's Department of Transport.

GLC — The Greater London Council.

Preface

'She was three years old and lived in decaying inner city housing where she was exposed to old leaded paint and to exhaust emissions from heavy passing traffic. When she was admitted to hospital she was stuperous, extremely pale, and her brain was swollen – a condition known as encephalopathy, the result of severe lead poisoning. I treated her with chelating agents and she recovered. I felt triumphant. I had made a good diagnosis. I had given the correct treatment and I saw the child getting better. Then when I told the mother that her daughter couldn't go back into that home she asked me "Where am I going to move? Every house on the block is the same". Confronted by those realities I began to realise that it is not enough just to give a drug. The disease is out there in the world, not just in the child.' *Dr. Herbert L. Needleman.*

THE WORD 'scandal' is defined in my dictionary as 'a stumbling block to faith . . . anything that brings discredit on the agent or agents by offending the moral feelings of the community'. That definition justifies the title of this book. The behaviour of the industries concerned with the addition of lead to petrol, and the failure of the authorities in many countries, including Britain, to act on the evidence that it is a hazard to health, should, in the case of the industries, offend the moral feelings of any caring community, and in the case of the authorities, undermine faith in their competence and integrity.

The book tells several stories:

There is the story of multi-national industries with enormous economic and political influence who have chosen to perpetuate a dangerous practice in order to protect profits; a practice they know threatens the health of the community, and particularly of children; a practice they ruthlessly defend in the face of widespread public concern.

There is the story of doctors and scientists who failed to appreciate the appalling risks inherent in adding lead to petrol, who consistently denied there was a problem until the evidence became overwhelming, and who, in many cases, even now prevaricate and delay while one generation of children after another become, in effect, guinea pigs for their research.

There is the story of public health authorities who have failed to perform their role adequately, let alone honourably; of how, when parents all over Britain combined together to fight for the health of their children, their main opponents became the very people who were appointed or elected to fulfil that public health role.

These interlocking stories raise a multitude of questions about industrial morality, environmental protection, the role of scientists in policy-making, and the need for and role of pressure groups in a so-called democratic society.

The 'plot' is easily described. Lead is a poison. It is added to petrol to boost the octane rating and is emitted from car exhausts in considerable quantities. It is then inhaled, picked up in dust, or absorbed via the food chain. Once inside the human system it is associated with a variety of health effects, and of these the most damaging are on the developing brains of young children. A fierce battle has taken place in the United States to protect children there. A Europe-wide campaign has been launched to persuade the EEC to fix a date for the phasing-out of lead in petrol. So far the biggest controversy has been in Britain where the authorities plan to reduce the maximum level of lead in petrol to 0.15 grams per litre by 1985. Opposition to this half-measure has been led by CLEAR, The Campaign for Lead-free Air.

In the first chapter we learn of the battle to reduce lead exposure in the United States and the endeavours by industrialists to frustrate legislative controls on their product.

We then explore the evidence that children's health is threatened by low level lead exposure, and the additional evidence that lead in petrol is a significant contributor to that exposure.

From there we look at the history of the controversy in Britain, the way the authorities took the decision in 1981 to keep lead in petrol, the success of the CLEAR campaign in arousing public concern about that decision, and the roles of the different protagonists in the battle that developed.

Finally, we look at how Britain and other European countries could move towards lead-free petrol, as Japan and the United States are well on the way to doing, and as Australia plans to do from the mid-Eighties.

Above all, however, the lead in petrol story represents a challenge to our priorities. What price do we put on health? How much do we value the purity of the air we breathe, the food we eat, and the water we drink? What do we care about most – the performance of our children or our cars? How much do we feel responsibility for the habitability of the planet we will leave for those to come?

I have no doubt where the priorities of most people lie. I have seen them reflected in the support for CLEAR throughout Britain. Our misfortune is that the institutions created to represent our concerns often have different priorities. Perhaps one message of this book is that we have to re-evaluate those institutions and determine how we can change them so that they reflect the long-term interests of people and their planet rather than vested interests and short-term compromise.

It is said that the price of liberty is eternal vigilance; in an age when the impact of technology on the whole planet is so considerable that we are in danger of undermining its very life-supporting qualities, we need to maintain vigilance and understand better the long-term implications for humanity of *all* that we do, and to implant within our authorities and bureaucracies a clear appreciation that there is a price for 'progress' that we are not always prepared to pay.

In his book *The Closing Circle*, the American environmentalist Barry Commoner wrote:

> Everywhere in the world there is evidence of a deep-seated failure in the effort to use the competence, the wealth, the power at human disposal for the maximum good of human beings. The environmental crisis is a major indication of this failure. . . . The environmental crisis is sombre evidence of an insidious fraud hidden in the vaunted product-ivity and wealth of modern, technology-based society. This wealth has been gained in a rapid short-term exploitation of the environmental system but it has blindly accumulated a debt to nature (in the form of environmental destruction in developed countries and of population pressure in the developing ones) – a debt so large and so pervasive that in the next generation it may, if unpaid, wipe out most of the wealth it has gained us.

Throughout the industrial revolution of the last century and the technological revolution of this century, we have systematically accumulated on the surface of our planet a highly dangerous neurotoxin, lead. Unlike many other environmental pollutants, lead is non-degradable. It does not disappear. It just accumulates and accumulates as we disperse more and more of it into our environment. It is probably impossible to evaluate accurately the damage that has already been done. And it is all too obvious that generations to come will inherit an appalling legacy of pollution unless we act now.

In the words of Dr. Needleman, quoted at the beginning of this introduction, 'The disease is out there in the world'. It is there because *we* have put it there, and it is within *our* power to control and reverse that process. We cannot start too soon.

VICTORY IN AMERICA ■

I.
How the environmentalists beat big business in the USA

RONALD REAGAN'S 1980 campaign to become President of the United States was not short of money. Big business, traditional supporters of the Republican Party, responded enthusiastically to Reagan's promise to 'get Washington off your backs'. The former film actor and Governor of California had, however, barely reached his desk in the Oval Office before those backers came looking for results. At the head of the queue was the petroleum industry. It demanded relief from what it considered unfair and unnecessary regulations controlling the addition of lead to petrol.

Reagan ordered his Vice-President, George Bush, to set up a special task force on regulatory relief and this duly published a 'hit-list' of regulations it claimed were 'burdensome, unnecessary, or counter-productive'. The lead phase-down programme was on the list. Bush passed responsibility for this to the Reagan hard-liner who had been appointed Administrator of the Environmental Protection Agency, Anne M. Gorsuch. There then began a battle between, on one side, the petroleum and lead industries, and on the other, environmentalists and public health organisations, over whether relaxation of controls on lead in petrol in the United States would damage the health of children. It was a crucial battle, not only for the US but for environmentalists all over the world, who had, up to this point, been able to quote the US as a precedent for the phasing out of lead in petrol and for whom a retreat by the Americans would be a major set-back.

The debate in the United States first took place in the early Seventies. Congress in 1970 passed a Clean Air Act to establish more stringent automobile emission standards. These were to become effective with 1975 model cars. After experimenting with a number of technological alternatives, all car manufacturers adopted catalytic converters to control such pollutants as carbon monoxide and hydrocarbons. The Environmental Protection Agency had been established in 1970 to consolidate in one agency much of the Federal authority and expertise to control pollution and other environmental threats. The Clean Air Act allowed the EPA to regulate fuel additives if this was necessary to allow the catalytic technology to work, and when it became clear that lead not only poisoned human beings, but also the catalysts, it was decided to prohibit the use of lead in petrol* in post-1975 cars.

However, Eric O. Stork, who was Deputy Assistant Administrator of the EPA from 1970–78 and directed the country's automobile emission control programme, is clear about the thinking at that time. He says:

> I have sometimes been asked if in the USA we took lead out of petrol for health reasons, or if we did it to make it possible to use catalytic converter exhaust emissions. The simple answer is that it was done for both reasons. . . . There is also a great deal of concern in our country about the adverse health effects of lead in the air, on the ground, and in the soil near roadways. For that reason we also established a programme that is phasing out the amount of lead allowed to be added to the petrol that still has some lead in it, i.e. the petrol that is used in older cars.

On May 30, 1975, the anti-knock industry, in the form of five petitioners, the Ethyl Corporation, PPG Industries, E. I. DuPont de Nemours & Company, NALCO Chemical Company, and the National Petroleum Refiners Association, took the Environmental Protection Agency to the US Court of Appeals in an attempt to have the reductions in the lead content of petrol over-turned. In the history of the lead-in-petrol debate, it was a crucial case, for to

---

* The Americans, of course, use the word 'gasoline'. For the sake of consistency I have altered it to 'petrol' throughout the book.

succeed the petitioners had to effectively challenge the EPA's self-interpreted freedom to act on the basis of risk rather than conclusive evidence, and then had to effectively challenge the evidence of risk itself. The court found that the EPA *had* acted within the law in assuming a precautionary role; thus, on public health issues, action could be justified on the basis of risk rather than conclusive evidence.

But was the population of the United States at risk from lead in petrol? The Court was in no doubt:

> From a vast mass of evidence the Administrator has concluded that the emission products of lead additives will endanger the public health. He has handled an extraordinarily complicated problem with great care and candour. The evidence did not always point in one direction and frequently, until EPA authorised research, there was no evidence at all. The Administrator reached his conclusion only after hearings spread over several months, considerations of thousands of pages of documents, publication of three health documents, three formal comment periods, and receipt of hundreds of comments. Each study was considered independently; its worth was assessed only after it was measured against any critical comments. From the totality of the evidence the Administrator concluded that regulation was warranted.
> In tracking his path through the evidence, we in our appellant role, have also considered separately each study and the objections petitioners make thereto. In no case have we found the Administrator's use of the evidence to be arbitrary or capricious. Having rejected the individual objections we also reject the overall claim of error. We find the Administrator's analysis of the evidence and assessment of the risks to be well within the flexibility allowed by the 'will danger' standard. Accordingly, we affirm his determination that lead emissions present a significant risk of harm to the health of urban populations, particularly to the health of city children.

The court also dealt with the question of whether the anti-lead measures were motivated by genuine concern for health, or to protect the catalysts:

> For years the lead anti-knock industry has refused to accept the developing evidence that lead emissions contribute significantly to the total human lead body burden. . . . However, Congress finally set up a legal mechanism by which that evidence could be weighed in a more objective tribunal. It gave the newly-created Environmental Protection Agency authority to control or prohibit the sale or manufacture of any fuel additive whose emission products 'endanger the public health or welfare . . .'. It is beyond question that the fuel additive Congress had in mind was lead.
> Given this mandate, the EPA published advance notice of proposed rule making. The Administrator announced he was considering

possible controls on lead additives in petrol, both *because of their possible dangers to health* and because of their incompatibility with the newly-developed catalytic converter emission control system.

So it was that in 1975 cars began to appear on the United States market equipped to run on lead-free petrol, and a wide range of brands of lead-free petrol began to appear at petrol stations all over the US. (It had, of course, already been on sale, for Amoco had marketed a lead-free brand of petrol for some years.) At the same time regulations began to come into effect limiting the lead that could be used in petrol for older cars.

Unfortunately, the United States failed to take a step that would have facilitated the growth of lead-free petrol. They did not intervene in any way to influence prices. The effect of this was a price difference between leaded and unleaded petrol. In 1982 this averaged five cents (or about threepence in English money). This had two negative effects: first, there was no incentive for owners of old cars to adapt them to lead-free petrol; second, a small proportion of owners of cars manufactured to run on lead-free petrol continued to use leaded petrol, unfortunately preferring the saving of five cents per gallon to the protection of children's health. (Leaded petrol causes no serious harm to a car manufactured to run on unleaded petrol; it only harms the catalytic converter, thus not only perpetuating emissions of lead but also of carbon monoxide and hydrocarbons). Nevertheless, by 1980 unleaded petrol represented well over half the petrol sold in the USA and by now it is about 60% and rising. As the pre-1975 generation of cars dies out, so the percentage of unleaded petrol used in the US will increase dramatically and ultimately, as in Japan, lead in petrol will virtually disappear.

At least that was the expectation until the election of Ronald Reagan and the instructions to Anne Gorsuch and the EPA to explore the possibility of abandoning or weakening the regulations. The effect of this would have been to allow the use of more lead in leaded petrol and thus to have increased lead emissions. Furthermore, it would possibly have enabled the manufacturers and retailers of leaded petrol to increase the price difference and thus encourage more drivers of post-1975 cars to break the law and abandon lead-free petrol. Ultimately it would threaten the ideal of lead-free petrol. The Presidential intervention on behalf of the industries represented more than just a test for the strength of the health evidence; it also represented a test of the genuine independence of the Environmental Protection Agency. Since 1970 it had become a substantial organisation with over 15,000 employees and more than 10 regional offices across the United States. It dealt with water quality, industrial and commercial waste, pesticides, toxic substances, air quality, noise, radiation, and described itself as protecting 'the country from being degraded, and our health threatened by a multitude of human activities initiated without regard to long-range effects upon the life-supporting properties, the economic uses, and the recreational value of air, land, and water'. Now it was headed by an Administrator, supported by her own appointees, under instructions from the White House to de-regulate where possible. So how would the EPA meet the test?

At first, it looked as if it would meet it badly. *Science* magazine reported that between May 1981 and March 1982 Gorsuch and her staff had private meetings with the refining and lead industries on 32 occasions without public observers present.

> The fact that the EPA met with refiners is not alarming in itself. . . . It is alarming that during all those months the EPA did not once seek information on new data becoming available on the toxic effects of lead.

Science magazine reported a meeting that took place on December 11, 1981, including Gorsuch, Larry Morgan from the staff of Senator Harrison Schmitt (a Republican Senator from New Mexico who was active lobbying for the refining industry in his state), two EPA officials, the Vice-President of Thriftway gasoline company of New Mexico, and two consulting attorneys for Thriftway, William Cockrell and Edward Shipper. The meeting was intended to persuade Gorsuch to allow Thriftway a special 'waiver' allowing the company to add more lead to petrol. *Science* reported that Gorsuch did not offer the waiver in writing but said she would not enforce the existing standards. A memo written by Shipper said in part:

> Gorsuch noted that EPA's lead phase-down regulations would probably be revised and perhaps even abolished during the course of the upcoming rule-making, in accordance with Vice-President Bush's expressed intentions. . . . We all thanked her and then left. . . . Larry Morgan, however, remained behind with Gorsuch momentarily. When he came out he told us that the Administrator explained to him that she couldn't actually tell us to go out and break the law, but that she hoped that we had gotten the message.

At first sight the battle seemed one-sided. There was the powerful petroleum industry, and especially the vociferous small refiners, who had been able to concentrate on the sale of leaded petrol with its price advantage in the market, and had the biggest vested interest in crushing the regulations. They had always been particularly effective in persuading State politicians to push their case in Washington. Then there was the lead industry, and the lead additive industry, each of them eager for greater sales. In a free enterprise country with an outstandingly free enterprise President and Administration, they could be forgiven for being confident of success.

In fact, it didn't work out like that at all. First there were leaks of the meetings between the EPA and the industries. This immediately put both parties on the defensive. Second, although Gorsuch and her own appointees were committed to an attempt to de-regulate lead in petrol, the old hands in the EPA, many of them with high ideals about the regulation of pollution, were not prepared to allow the Agency to be discredited. They influenced events both by battling hard within the Agency, and by being prepared to leak material outside. Then there was the campaign by the environmentalists, including the Environmental Defense Fund (whose brilliant specialist on toxic pollution, Ellen Silbergeld, co-ordinated much of the scientific protest), the Natural Resources Defense Fund (led by their determined lawyer, Eric Goldstein), and outspoken scientists like Dr. Herbert Needleman, prominent researcher into the ill effects of lead, Dr. Ed Groth, Director of Public Service projects at the Consumers Union, and others. Their main ally on Capitol Hill was the Democratic Congressman from Connecticut, Toby Moffett.

The environmentalists had powerful allies in the media. As soon as the news broke, a number of leading newspapers attacked the EPA's manoeuvres. *Science* magazine described hearings chaired by Moffett as 'a public relations disaster for the EPA and the refineries'. *The New York Times* attacked Gorsuch in a leader:

> What civilised Government would want to take the risk of endangering its children's minds, even for a far greater gain than is at stake here?

The *Washington Post* reported that the EPA was:

> trying to extricate itself from what has become another Agency public relations fiasco. . . . The EPA has to figure out how to deal with two studies it has commissioned and its staff analyses that all concluded that hundreds of thousands of children could get lead poisoning if the standards were weakened.

One EPA source told the *Washington Post*:

> They (the Reagan Administration) couldn't have picked a worse thing to target. It has been studied just about more than any other toxin and relaxing lead standards would put us in favour of harming the health of hundreds of thousands of children at a time when the EPA is trying

to fight an image that it is becoming soft on polluting industries and dangerous substances.

The influential syndicated columnist Jack Anderson then joined the row with a column read by millions of Americans stating:

> Incredibly, the Reagan Administration appears willing to risk the health of hundreds of thousands of anonymous pre-schoolers, just so the oil companies can make a few bucks.

Moffett chaired a hearing on Capitol Hill that exposed the manoeuvrings that had taken place between Gorsuch and her appointees and the refiners. He forced a further two days of hearings on the health and scientific evidence, and these proved disastrous for

---

'I am writing to you in my capacity as a physician. As Chief of Haematology in the Division of Paediatrics of a large city hospital in New York, I have the painful daily experience of witnessing the unnecessary and often irreparable damage produced by lead to the immature brain and body of children . . .

'My clinical experience and my research work lead to the inexorable conclusion that screening of children after they have been exposed to lead is to public health the equivalent of closing the stable door after the horse has bolted . . .

'The urgency of decreasing the blood lead level of children is pointed out by the fact that modern techniques show adverse effects at blood lead levels much lower than previously thought even in the so-called "normal" range. Recent studies have shown clear impairment of neurological and physiological function in children with blood lead levels in the upper limit of the "normal" range. Bio-chemical evidence of damage by lead can be demonstrated at blood lead levels frighteningly low. These findings have been considered in the many comments by the lead industry and its hired consultants as meaningless laboratory tests. This view by those who have a vested interest in maintaining high concentrations of lead in the air has, unfortunately, from a point of view of public health, very little scientific value . . .

'It has been obvious, through these months, that enormous pressures have been put on the Environmental Protection Agency by those groups who have large economical interests to avoid any reduction in the present levels of exposure to lead. It is certainly necessary that the EPA hear and consider the comments of the involved industry to avoid a capriciously restrictive standard. On the other hand, the Agency should fulfil its role as the protector of the health of these most sensitive citizens, the children, especially of the poor, who can mobilise in their defence only a minute fraction of the resources available to large corporations.' *Letter from Sergio Piomelli, MD, Professor of Pediatrics, Director of Pediatric Haematology, New York University Medical Center, to the Administrator, Environmental Protection Agency.*

---

the EPA. Needleman described his studies and told the hearing:

> I believe that such a step, if taken, would go directly against the grain of modern public health thinking, would put thousands of children back at risk of impaired brain function and would cast justifiable doubt on the nation's commitment to the public health of our young citizens. . . . The question of lead's hazards to children no longer needs debate. Animal studies and careful clinical studies with human beings have demonstrated this to the satisfaction of all but those who have a vested financial interest in the sale of lead products. . . . Airborne lead, over 90% of it from petrol, contributes substantially to the exposure of children. When lead in petrol has been decreased, blood levels have dropped consistently. The setting of a lead standard and the lowering of air lead levels in communities has been one of the most crucial public health actions of the decade. I believe it will be a tragic mistake, one whose impact will be felt by our children and children yet to be born, to relax the phase-down of lead in petrol.

Ed Groth, who had been a staff member of the Environmental Studies Board of the National Academy of Science's National Research Council and had directed the study by the Committee on Lead in the Human Environment whose report was published in 1980, reminded the hearing that the report had . . .

> concluded quite unequivocally that the levels of lead to which we are exposed are unacceptably high. The report stresses particularly the hazards of lead levels to many thousands of inner city children who are routinely exposed. The Committee recommended that more extensive efforts be made to remove sources of exposure that affect children, and also that a serious effort be made to lower the general population's exposure to lead.

Groth went on:

> The EPA's reasoning is flawed in all its particulars:
> EPA presumes that a short-term *increase* in lead emissions from automobiles would have no unacceptable health impact. In fact, however, the health impact of amounts of lead already in the environment is presently unacceptable; to permit the release of *more* lead into the air can only exacerbate an already intolerable hazard.
> EPA's assertion that the lead-in-petrol standards deal with a source of short-term air quality impacts is scientifically unsupportable. Lead emitted to the air ends up in the soil, in dust, and in the food chain. Through all manner of complex environmental transfers, lead from the original petrol source reaches children. Exposure to petrol lead in dust and soil is a persisting long-term problem that will remain for decades after the last tankful of leaded petrol is ever pumped.
> Lead in petrol is indisputably a major source of exposure. Although

precise estimates of the quantitative contribution of any one source are scientifically untenable, the need to protect children from toxic effects of lead is inextricably tied to a need to continue to reduce the pollution of the environment by lead from motor vehicle exhaust.

The industries fought back. They claimed the proposed change would have an insignificant impact on children with high blood lead levels and would not cause them any harm. The phase-down would have 'no adverse health effects, it would have important energy savings and economic benefits'. They called a number of scientists to support their case.

The debate extended into late May. At that point John Bell, a senior official within the United States Office of Consumer Affairs, sent a memo to his own Administrator. This, too, was leaked. In it he said:

Although you have stated a policy of non-intervention for this office, I believe that EPA's proposal to weaken the levels of toxic lead in petrol raises such serious health hazards for susceptible population groups, especially children in congested urban areas, that it is imperative to appraise you of the current status of this proposal and recommend that you take positive action regarding the matter.

EPA's proposal has generated strong adverse reactions for a very simple reason: lead is a toxic metal that can cause, among other things, brain damage and death. Infants and growing children are far more susceptible to heavy metal poisoning than are adults. It is known that the threshold level for cell damage in children is extremely low, although there is not total agreement on how low that threshold is. Thus, there is considerable doubt whether EPA's existing lead standards protect human health. A growing body of evidence indicates there may be *no* safe minimum levels for children. . . .

In addition to the human suffering that would likely be caused by weakening the lead standards, adverse economic impacts would be staggering. Dr. Joel Schwartz of EPA's Office of Policy and Resource Management, concluded that eliminating the lead standard would save industry about $100 million a year. However, he estimated that it would cost $140 million–$1.4 billion to treat the additional 200,000–500,000 children that would get lead poisoning. . . .

Recommendation: Since there is no rational or defensible medical, economic or political basis to support weakening the existing lead in petrol standard, it is recommended that you make the dangers of lead poisoning known, inside the White House and externally. Once people understand the real danger of toxic metal poisoning, I believe they can only reach one decision – to oppose weakening EPA's existing lead standard and to re-evaluate the existing standard. This could be the most significant position you take in your office in terms of the health of children and consumers.

Whether or not the Office of Consumer Affairs acted on this strongly-worded advice, the EPA was receiving equally outspoken advice from within its own office, notably from Dr. Joel Schwartz. He circulated a document within the EPA to support the evidence of health damage at low levels of exposure. As the Bell memo indicated, Schwartz suggested that not only was the health case proven, but that you could put a price on the health damage caused to children and it was greater than the cost of further reducing lead in petrol.

About this time the Center for Disease Control and the National Center for Health Statistics demonstrated that environmental lead from petrol had dropped from 190,000 tonnes to 90,000 tonnes between 1976 and 1980, and that correspondingly, the overall mean blood level of the US population had fallen by 36.7%. As a result, Congressman Berkley Bedell of Iowa moved a resolution opposing the EPA relaxation of lead standards in the House of Representatives:

> The studies by the Center for Disease Control point to a close relationship between the amount of lead in petrol and the concentration of lead in our bodies. Consequently, it would be a great mistake to thwart the progress we have made in fighting lead poisoning in the United States by increasing the lead content of petrol.

By now it was clear that the EPA would have to make a choice: on the one hand, it could please the President and big business by reducing controls on lead in petrol, or, on the other, it could perform the role of an environmental protection agency and insist on environmental protection. The EPA passed its test. In late July 1982, Kathleen Bennett, Assistant Administrator for Air, Noise and Radiation, advised Gorsuch that 'relaxation of the regulations is not warranted. In fact, new studies support the concept that lead emissions should be minimised'.

Newspapers reported:

> The EPA in a dramatic policy reversal is expected to announce that it will abandon efforts to weaken restrictions and will tighten up instead. . . .

'The Bush Commission would be well advised to zero in on those regulations that are truly burdensome, unnecessary, and counterproductive. Judged by these standards, lead phase-down ought to be one of the first to go.' *Oil and Gas Journal.*

'Had we known in 1972 what we know now, I believe we would have banned lead in gasoline completely over five years.' *Dr. Joel Schwartz of the Environmental Protection Agency.*

So it was that the EPA posted into the Federal Register its proposals:

> EPA determined that rescinding or relaxing the present lead standard would result in an increase of lead emissions to the atmosphere, that environmental lead exposure continues to be a national health concern, and that there is no new information that would lead EPA to determine that continued control of lead in petrol is not appropriate.

It proposed tighter controls that would further reduce lead in petrol.

The Agency said it had received over 1,100 written comments and oral testimony by over 110 witnesses, and, reviewing the history of the issue, confirmed that health effects were a key factor in the beginning of phasing out of lead in petrol in the early Seventies.

> The Agency recognised that the extent of the contribution of lead in petrol to the lead exposure problem in this country was controversial and complex. EPA nevertheless concluded that in its judgement there were sufficient health-based concerns to initiate a regulatory programme to reduce the use of lead in petrol. The lead phase-down programme was based on the premise that petrol lead emissions should be controlled to the extent possible.
>
> The general findings leading to the Agency's *initial* (1970) decision to regulate lead usage in petrol (were):
>
> (a) Environmental lead exposure is a major health problem in this country. A small but significant proportion of the urban adult population and up to 25% of the children in urban areas are over-exposed to lead.
>
> (b) The lead exposure problem is caused by a combination of sources . . . including food, water, air, leaded paint and dust.
>
> (c) It is extremely difficult to determine what percentage of the problem each separate environmental factor contributes.
>
> (d) Since the sources are additive and their importance varies considerably, it is difficult to determine what impact would be achieved by a partial or total reduction of lead from any source.
>
> (e) A reduction of lead in all sources would substantially improve the situation.
>
> (f) Lead in petrol is a source of air and dust lead which can be readily and significantly reduced in comparison to other sources.
>
> (g) Lead from petrol accounts for over 90% of the airborne lead and combined with lead from stationary sources and deteriorating lead-based paint, causes high lead levels in dirt and dust.
>
> (h) Lead in petrol is the most ubiquitous source of lead in dust, dirt, and air.
>
> (i) Human exposure resulting from lead in petrol comes from inhalation of airborne lead and from ingestion of dirt and dust contaminated by fallout from airborne lead.

(j) Since exposure to lead among the general population is widespread, it is reasonable that efforts be made to reduce preventable sources of lead exposure, including lead emissions resulting from lead in petrol.

The EPA insert in the Federal Register then went on to discuss the up-to-date health evidence:

The majority of the (1982) comments emphatically rejected the proposition that lead was no longer a public health problem. Sixty-four comments were received from the professional health community and academia. Sixty of these opposed any loosening of the lead standard, and many suggested that tighter controls would be desirable. Thirty-two comments were received from local and state government. All of these supported retention of the current standard to protect their children's health. Most of the commentators pointed to previous studies, as well as their own experiences to demonstrate that lead has an adverse effect on people at very low dosages, and that the more the problem is studied, the lower the acceptable level of lead becomes. They concluded that protection of public health and welfare demands that all reasonable steps be taken to eliminate lead from the environment.

The EPA then went on to examine all of the evidence on the relationship between body lead burdens and lead in petrol and concluded:

On balance, after reviewing all of the studies mentioned and the record of this proceeding, EPA is persuaded that environmental exposure to lead from petrol is a significant contributor to total lead exposure of the population.

Thus, the EPA concluded:

There are insufficient health grounds upon which a rescission or relaxation of the lead phase-down programme can be based. The rationale for the original decision by EPA to regulate the use of lead in petrol has been re-examined and no new information has been submitted which would warrant a shift in the original rationale to control lead in petrol. Insufficient evidence has been presented to show that a health problem related to environmental exposure to lead, particularly in urban areas, does not continue to exist. Nor has it been shown that petrol lead is not a major source of lead exposure via inhalation of air lead or ingestion of dirt or dust lead.

Environmental and public health groups had barely the time to open the first bottle of celebratory champagne before the White House stepped in. The Office of Management and Budget (OMBE) in the President's office asked the EPA to postpone its new regulation and reconsider its 'appropriateness'.

Science magazine reported:

> The EPA faces a dilemma. One EPA official says the Agency has three choices: accept the changes the White House wants, even though they are not based on new health or economic data; negotiate a compromise; or thank the White House for its comments and proceed to adopt the rules as written. The last option may be legally permissible, but politically chancy for the officials who will make the decision.

By now, however, it was clear to the EPA that the unpopularity they would suffer in the White House would be more tolerable than the alternative of widespread public protest, let alone having to abandon the function and ideals of the Agency. It therefore found itself in a fight with the White House, but finally in November confirmed its policy. As a last-ditch manoeuvre, the small refiners went to court to seek an injunction to postpone implementation of the tougher regulations, but the court rejected their appeal. The environmentalists had won.

The implications of this story for those countries, like Britain, embroiled in debates about lead in petrol, are threefold:

First, it cannot be over-emphasised that the 1982 US debate was about health alone. The question was: did lead from petrol threaten health, and if so, should the lead phase-down programme be continued? The US answer was that it should not only be continued but accelerated. Such was the strength of the evidence of health hazard.

Second, the EPA began the exercise actually prejudiced towards relaxation of the regulations, but on the evidence of the relationship between lead in petrol and body lead burdens had no alternative but to reverse its own momentum and ultimately fight the White House itself. Such was the strength of the environmental pollution case.

Third, it demonstrated that no matter how powerful a polluting industry may be, if the public, and its watchdogs, the consumer, environmental and public health agencies, care enough and fight hard enough, the public interest can prevail.

There is still lead in petrol in the United States, but over the years it will gradually disappear. The Americans have set a standard that the rest of the world can and should follow. That they have done so is a tribute to the courage, scientific brilliance and social responsibility of those environmentalists who took on big business and won.

THE THREAT TO HEALTH

2.
Children at risk

Give to men who are old and rougher
The things that little children suffer
And let's keep bright and undefiled
The young years of the little child.
John Masefield

NO-ONE – not even the lead industry – denies that lead is toxic.
To be toxic is to act as a poison. Lead, being a neurotoxin, is a brain
poison. Excessive exposure to lead (i.e. around 80 ug/dl) can cause
severe behavioural disturbances, abdominal pain, anaemia, nerve
palsy, epilepsy, convulsions, paralysis, coma, and even death. This
is known as 'classical' or 'clinical lead poisoning' and *is not the subject
of this book*, for the lead-in-petrol controversy centres on two basic
questions:

1   Is there danger to human beings, especially children, from
     much lower levels of exposure to lead – i.e. levels that in
     developed countries are now considered normal?
2   Is lead in petrol a major contributor to that exposure?
     Clearly there is no need to answer the second question if the

answer to the first is negative. Before we come to the lead-in-petrol question, therefore, we have to establish just what is at stake.

Children are at least four to five times more vulnerable to the ill effects of lead than adults. This is explained by the Canadian scientist J. F. Jaworski in a report to the National Research Council of Canada:

Children are a special case. They are more susceptible to the adverse effects of lead than are adults for a number of reasons. Lead crosses the placental barrier with ease. Thus exposure may occur during prenatal development, a stage especially prone to the effects of toxic chemicals. Young children have a higher rate of lead absorption from the gut (45–50 per cent, or almost five times that for adults) and this may be increased by calcium or iron deficiency or even by high levels of dietary milk. A greater fraction of the body content of lead in children is found in the soft tissues in a highly mobile form (4–9 times that of adults) which is toxic to tissues. Children have higher metabolic rates than do adults and rapidly growing tissue is often more easily affected by toxic substances than is slower growing tissue. On a dose-per-body-weight basis, children absorb more lead than do adults, not only because of their higher metabolic rate (higher rate of food utilisation and higher rate of lead absorption) but also because of mouthing of non-food items which may be contaminated with lead from airborne fallout or paint.

Taken as a whole, the evidence indicates that at everyday levels of lead exposure, especially in towns and cities, children are at risk of . . .

● reduced IQ
● learning difficulties because they are more easily distracted or frustrated
● behavioural problems
● hyperactivity

In other words, they are at risk of not achieving their full potential in life.

Lead has been added to petrol for many years, as it had been added to paint and used in water pipes, before the first studies began to appear in the scientific literature indicating permanent neurotoxic effects at much lower levels of lead exposure than those likely to cause clinical lead poisoning. Even then the medical profession and public health authorities were reluctant to respond to them.

(There are, of course, plenty of precedents for this inertia. Take asbestos. The International Agency for Research on Cancer said in 1977: 'By the time the cancer potential of asbestos had been recognised and defined (1935–60), asbestos had penetrated much of modern industry, and indeed, modern society, with thousands of products being manufactured and utilised throughout the world and in circumstances that we now understand were inadequate for the control of occupational diseases including cancer. As a result, we are now faced with a double dilemma, of how to deal with the consequences of previous inattention and error, in terms of human diseases, and of how to avoid further exposure which could produce disease in the future.' Even more disturbing is that we don't know how many other hazards to health already exist, their effects as yet undetected. Take chemicals: Eric Eckholm in his book *Down to Earth* reports that 'Synthetic chemicals permeate modern life. At least 55,000 are produced commercially, and a thousand new ones are manufactured each year. In developed countries people are exposed to chemicals in the air they breathe, the water they drink, the food they eat, the drugs they take, and the products they handle each day at home and at work. . . . Modern chemicals have undoubtedly created benefits. But an unknown proportion cause cancer, birth defects, or other human ills, or damage plants and animals. Having accepted the proliferation of chemicals without much control in the past, societies now face the expensive and complex tasks of identifying those that are dangerous and then deciding what to do about them.')

Lead compounds exist in two forms. The two petrol additives, tetramethyl lead and tetraethyl lead, are both *organic lead* compounds. These can be absorbed through the skin and penetrate easily to nerve tissue, including the brain. They are therefore extremely neurotoxic. The lethal dose of tetraethyl lead is one quarter of a gram and that makes it 10 times as toxic as inorganic lead. *Inorganic lead* is used in paint, plumbing, lead solders, etc. Most of the lead emitted from car exhausts has also by then become inorganic and all the studies with children measure the level of inorganic lead in the blood-stream.

Children absorb inorganic lead by breathing it into their lungs and by ingestion (normal eating and drinking, and fortuitous ingestion of lead-rich dust, dirt, soil, paint, etc.) A typical urban child not exposed to any special source of lead intoxication will probably have a blood lead level below 30 ug/dl. Children with blood lead levels above 30 ug/dl are probably exposed to extra sources of pollution, such as plumbosolvent water supplies, flakes of leaded paint, lead smelters, etc.

Dr. Robin Russell Jones, CLEAR's adviser on lead and health, explains what happens once lead is inside the human system:

> The lead is carried in the blood stream mainly by red cells. An equilibrium is established between the level of lead in blood and the level of lead in soft tissues, i.e. muscle, brain, liver, spleen, kidneys, etc. Some of the lead is also excreted so there is a balance between the amount absorbed from the lungs and the gastrointestinal tract, and the

amount excreted. Lead is an accumulative poison within the body and although the level of lead in blood may remain fairly constant throughout life, the level of lead in soft tissue increases during early life and the level of lead in bone continues to accumulate throughout life.

It is sometimes said that this lead is of no importance since it is not biologically available, i.e. it has disappeared into the skeleton and does not pose any sort of health threat. This is not so. If a lead worker has been exposed to excessive quantities of lead and he is then removed from his source of exposure his blood lead level will remain elevated for many years due to the recycling of lead from his skeleton. The effects of lead within the human system are extremely complex and still not completely understood. However, lead does have a very profound influence on a number of biological systems apart from the brain. Thus, one of the enzymes which forms the blood pigment haem is inhibited by lead at levels of 15 ug/dl and below. This enzyme is known as amino-levulinic acid dehydratase and a rise in the level of delta amino-levulinic acid is one of the best documented effects of lead at low dosage. Lead also has the ability to inhibit or influence the activity of many enzymes which are involved in normal brain functioning. Chemicals transmitting nerve impulses into the brain are profoundly affected by lead at very low doses. These effects have been mainly demonstrated by animal experiments.

Because lead has been shown to affect so many neurotransmitters and so many biological systems within the human body, the effects of lead in the brain are liable to be panoramic, i.e. it won't just affect one aspect of neurological function. It will probably affect them all: IQ, behaviour, memory, reaction times, personality, etc.

It is probably because of the immense complexity of lead's effects on the human brain that there is still so much debate about what these exactly are. Sometimes I feel it would be simpler to reduce the debate to what lead doesn't do.

The Canadian, J. F. Jaworski, also described in his report the effect of lead on the brain and nervous system:

Lead affects both the central and peripheral nervous systems of mammals. The young are especially susceptible because, compared with adults, they appear to have no barrier to lead entry to the nervous system and their nervous systems are still in the developmental stage. Damage to the nervous system is usually partly or fully irreversible because repair processes are very slow or non-existent. In the brain lead tends to concentrate in the hippocampus (a structure which has been implicated in the control of emotional behaviour, learning and memory) and in the amygdala (also involved in the expression of behavioural traits). Thus, it is not surprising that degenerative changes in behaviour, learning, motor-functioning (hand-eye co-ordination) and memory are amongst the first effects of lead observable, especially in children. Furthermore, studies with rats indicate that parental exposure to elevated levels of lead before mating adversely affected the learning ability of the offspring. The effects of paternal and maternal exposure were additive.

Adverse biochemical changes (impaired glucose metabolism, inhibition of adenyl cyclase) begin to occur at brain lead levels currently observed in the general population. A growing body of information points to hyperactivity as well as the decreased cognitive, verbal and perceptual ability, in some children, as the result of moderate increases in lead absorption. This is supported by experiments with rats and sheep.

Mental retardation is a recognised result of overt or acute lead

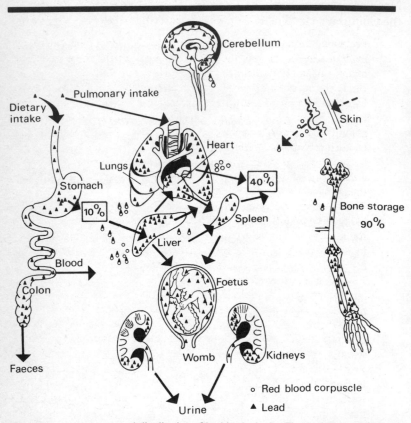

Figure 1   UPTAKE AND and distribution of lead in the body. The dynamic equilibrium between lead intake and excretion. Nearly all ingested material is excreted with only around 10–20% of ingested material absorbed. This is then distributed to the soft tissues with around 9 ug daily in adults being stored in bone. The principal mode of excretion is through the kidneys. The greatest concentration of lead will be found in the bone. All soft tissues including the foetus have similar concentrations within them. Source: Dr. Michael Moore, CLEAR Symposium, May 1982

poisoning in young children. Furthermore, about 10% of children with high levels of lead but with no overt signs of lead toxicity later exhibited varying degrees of retardation.

The Evidence of Risk

One study that was more instrumental than any other in forcing the medical and scientific world to take the issue seriously, was by Herbert Needleman and colleagues, in the United States, first reported in the *New England Journal of Medicine* in 1979. Dr. Needleman, now Associate Professor of Psychiatry and Pediatrics at the Children's Hospital of Pittsburgh, described his work to me:

Previous studies in this area were criticised and often flawed by inadequacies in the way the research was executed. There were four main problems with them:
First, the markers of earlier lead exposure were poor. Most studies had relied on blood lead to classify exposure but this is a short-term marker because it can sometimes return to normal after a child stops assimilating large quantities of the metal. Thus, blood lead levels can be normal while tissue leads are high.
Second, measure of the outcome of studies were often insensitive . . . we really needed sensitive measures to detect impairment that was less than obvious.
Third, there was often inadequate attention to non-lead variables likely to confound the effect of lead on the outcome. It was necessary to identify and control for other variables such as family background, including parental intelligence, environmental conditions, and socio-economic status. Medical history was often neglected.
Finally, many of the studies were biased in the selection. A study that aims to provide conclusions applicable to the community as a whole must draw its sample from a representative population.
In 1975 we collected teeth from over 3,000 first and second grade children attending ordinary, non-remedial classes from two primarily white, working-class towns adjacent to Boston, Massachusetts. Previously, teeth had been shown to accurately mark past exposure to lead well after exposure had ended. Children whose dentine lead levels were in the highest 10% (greater than 20 ppm) were classified as having high lead levels, and those in the lowest 10% (less than 10 ppm) were classified as low lead. Those children who had been born at term, had no significant head injuries or neurological diseases, had never been known to have excess lead exposure, and spoke English as a first language at home, were invited to participate in the neuro-psychological follow-up study.
To evaluate the selection bias we compared the children included in the study with children not participating on distribution of lead levels and teacher ratings on an 11-item classroom behaviour scale. The

included children did not differ from the excluded children in either dimension.

While the child was being tested, the mother filled out a lengthy questionnaire evaluating 39 non-lead covariates. She also took a brief IQ test. When high and low lead subjects were compared on these covariates, only five showed a difference of any significance. The children were then given an extensive neurobehavioural set of tests in fixed order by psychometricians who were unaware of the children's dentine levels. They evaluated the children on psychometric intelligence, concrete operational intelligence, academic achievement, auditory and language processing, visual motor coordination, attentional performance, and motor coordination using standard scientific test procedures and some novel tests designed for the study.

We attempted to secure a teacher's rating on each child who gave a tooth. This was based on an 11-item questionnaire.

In the data analysis we employed an analysis of covariance with lead as the main effect. The mother's age at the time of the child's birth, the mother's education, family size, the father's socio-economic status, and parental IQ were the five variables entered into the model and controlled.

To put it simply, Needleman and his colleagues had created a study whereby it was possible to compare IQ and behaviour of children with high and low lead levels whilst taking into account other factors that could influence the result.

The Needleman behavioural study above (and in figure 1 on page 22) compared teacher's ratings on 11 factors for 2,146 children with their tooth lead levels and showed a clear association between negative ratings and higher lead levels. The teachers who did the ratings were not informed of the children's lead levels.

The Yule and Lansdown 1981 study (figure 2 on page 23) replicated in Britain the Needleman findings to a remarkable extent.

The full 11 questions were:

1   Is this child easily distracted during his/her work?
2   Can he/she persist with a task for a reasonable amount of time?
3   Can this child work independently and complete assigned tasks with minimal assistance?
4   Is his/her approach to tasks disorganised (constantly misplacing pencils, books, etc.)?
5   Do you consider this child hyperactive?
6   Is he/she over-excitable and impulsive?
7   Is he/she easily frustrated by difficulties?
8   Is he/she a daydreamer?
9   Can he/she follow simple directions?
10 Can he/she follow a sequence of directions?
11 In general, is this child functioning as well in the classroom as other children his/her own age?

And what was the result? *The children with low lead levels performed better on 10 of the 11 items.* Lead was seen to be associated with deficits in IQ, verbal IQ, auditory processing and reaction time under varying intervals of delay. The teachers rated the children with high lead levels over twice as frequently negative on each item they evaluated.

In addition, we cross-tabulated all 2,146 children on whom we had a teacher's rating scale and at least one dentine level. The subjects were classified into six groups according to dentine lead level, and the percentage of negative reports for each item calculated. We found that the higher lead levels in teeth were consistently related to negative ratings of the children.

No-one has since been able to seriously fault the Needleman study. Professor Michael Rutter, who surveyed the evidence on 'impaired cognitive/behavioural function' for the DHSS working party on lead (the Lawther Committee), was critical of most of the other research in the area, but acknowledged that . . .

The study by Needleman et al. provides the most impressive evidence to date on the possible damaging effects of raised lead levels in the range usually previously considered harmless and which are found in some 20% of children in the general population. There are a number of important questions and reservations about the study and the inferences to be drawn from them, but *none of these are sufficient to invalidate the findings*

Later in his report to Lawther, Rutter said:

Altogether, this seems to be a well planned, detailed, systematic and well analysed study – probably the best available to date – and clearly the results demand serious consideration.

Two crucial points:

Firstly, one cannot over-emphasise that Needleman met the essential test of allowing for other explanations (39 of them) before reaching his conclusions.

Secondly, the increase in a child's problems in direct relation to the level of lead in teeth (as can be clearly seen in figure 2) indicates dose-dependency. This implies more than just an association between high lead levels and mental impairment – it is significant evidence of cause.

Nevertheless, even a study as respected as Needleman's had to be replicated before other scientists would accept it as a basis for action. This is the significance of the work of Drs. William Yule and Richard Lansdown and colleagues in London published in 1981–2.

Yule and Lansdown had been members of the Lawther Committee and subsequent to its work were commissioned to undertake research to establish whether the Needleman findings could be replicated in Britain. They compared the blood lead levels of 166 Greenwich school children with their intelligence and performance, dividing them into children with blood-lead levels of 12 ug/dl and below, and those with 13 ug/dl up to 32 ug/dl. It should be stressed that every one of the 166 children had blood lead levels below the safety threshold of 35 ug/dl endorsed by the Lawther Committee and sustained by Whitehall.

The results showed that *the children with the higher lead levels (but all below the official safety threshold) had an average IQ deficit of seven points.* Even more disturbing, their behavioural analysis on the same 11-issue basis replicated Needleman's findings.

While Yule and Lansdown emphasised that further research was necessary, they stated that their work indicated a dose-response-relationship between increasing lead levels and an increased likelihood that teachers would record deviant behaviour:

> We would claim that with our broad replication of Needleman et al's findings and their extension to relating lead levels to activity levels . . . we have provided hard evidence of an association between increasing

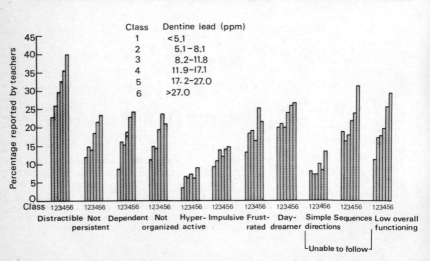

Figure 2   THE CHART produced by Needleman et al. in 1979 to demonstrate the relationship between lead in teeth of children and behavioural and educational difficulties

lead levels and interference with focusing attention and increased activity. The studies point to low but statistically significant (i.e. real) correlations between lead levels and IQ. In the context of IQ, low correlations are more believable than large ones.

By comparing figures 2 and 3 we can see only too clearly that Yule and Lansdown in their study confirmed Needleman's findings.

Yule and Lansdown were, at the time this book was being written, undertaking further research and 'controlling' for social factors and parental intelligence. During the autumn of 1982 it became known that the Medical Research Council had received an advance report from them on a further study in the Greenwich area. Although most of the children came from middle class backgrounds, about fifty came from working class backgrounds. Evidence of ill effects was found within that sub-group at levels as low as 10 ug/dl but there was little evidence of such effects in the middle class children. This second study is likely to add to confusion on the issue generally, but the findings indicate the possibility that lead's effects are maximised in situations where counterbalancing effects, such as good nutrition, parental motivation, etc., are deficient. There is therefore reason to believe that working class children are not only more exposed to lead, but because of their inadequate diet, they are also less protected. These also tend to be the children most exposed

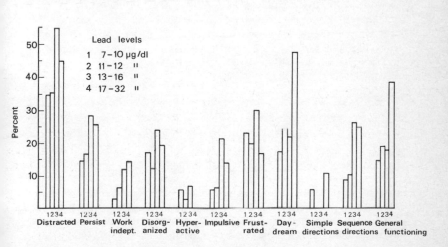

Figure 3   RESULTS OF a study conducted in Britain by Yule and Lansdown, 1981, which replicates the Needleman findings.

to lead. As far back as July 1978 the *New Scientist* had argued that lead pollution was partly a class issue:

> Airborne lead pollution is not democratic. It falls more heavily on the heads of some communities than on others. The children who may suffer excess lead pollution from car exhausts are those living near main roads in the big cities. Broadly speaking, these are working class children of parents not skilled in the arts of bringing pressure on authorities.

Further support for the Needleman and Yule and Lansdown studies came from Professor Gerhard Winneke and colleagues at the Medical Institute of Environmental Hygiene, University of Dusseldorf, who established a difference of between 5 and 7 IQ points between children with high and low lead levels. Winneke concluded that his 'data clearly supports the findings of Needleman et al'. Further work by Winneke confirmed the association between tooth lead levels and psychological malfunction. Professor Rutter, summing up the Winneke research at the CLEAR symposium, stated:

> Three aspects of Winneke's research warrant special emphasis. First, the associations on some of the key measures remained even after possibly confounding social variables had been fully taken into account (indeed, this is particularly striking as there are reasons for supposing that there may have been some over-correction through the use of school variables that will have included variance due to differences in the children's behaviour and intelligence prior to school entry). Second, these apply to lead levels below the supposedly safe limit of 35 ug/dl. Third, the differential pattern of findings after controlling for confounding variables has implications for the possible mechanisms by which raised lead levels predispose to psychological impairment.

During 1982 Dr. David Otto, research psychologist with the US Environmental Protection Agency, came to Britain to describe research he and scientists had undertaken at the Biological Sciences Research Center of the University of North Carolina. They had produced evidence that lead causes changes in the electrical activity

---

'The cognitive deficits which have been found have usually been of the order of 3 to 5 points, and it has been argued that a 5-point difference is so trivial in its effects that it can be safely ignored. That is a totally fallacious arguent . . . a drop of five points in mean IQ . . . for any population must necessarily result in more than a 2-fold increase in the percentage of individuals with an IQ below 70, i.e. a doubling of the number of mentally retarded children.' *Professor Michael Rutter*.

Per cent 'deviant' at two blood-lead levels

	Item	Blood-lead level 7–12 ug/dl %	13–32 ug/dl %
1	Restless	26.8	33.3
2	Truants	6.1	0
3	Squirmy	13.4	32.1
4	Destroys	3.7	9.5
5	Fights	6.1	20.2
6	Not liked	11.0	16.7
7	Worried	30.5	35.7
8	Solitary	19.5	26.2
9	Irritable	8.5	15.5
10	Miserable	17.1	16.7
11	Twitches	6.1	9.5
12	Sucks thumb	1.2	8.3
13	Bites nails	3.7	11.9
14	Absent	14.6	13.1
15	Disobedient	9.8	21.4
16	Can't settle	14.6	25.0
17	Fearful	28.0	35.7
18	Fussy	17.1	15.5
19	Lies	8.5	16.7
20	Steals	1.2	6.0
21	Inert	9.8	20.2
22	Aches	13.4	10.7
23	Tears	11.0	4.8
24	Stutters	6.1	9.5
25	Resentful	11.0	15.5
26	Bullies	8.5	14.3

THE TABLE above from the Yule and Lansdown study in Greenwich illustrates the tendency to 'deviancy' at higher levels of lead.

of children's brains, even when it is present in only small quantities. Furthermore, he indicated that there is no burden of lead so small as to produce no effect on the brain's electrical activity, further undermining the concept of a safety threshold.

Soon after (in May 1982) the proceedings of the National Academy of Science in the United States published details of a biochemical study showing that even so-called 'normal' blood-lead levels can inhibit the production of haemoglobin, the essential oxygen-carrying molecule of the blood.

Dr. Bernard Davidow and colleagues at the New York Medical

Center measured the amounts of haemoglobin precursor known as red-blood-cell protoporphyrin in the blood of 2,000 New York children and compared it with their blood lead concentrations.

They confirmed early work showing that the precursor concentration rose very rapidly (exponentially) among children with high blood lead levels, indicating that haemoglobin production was being blocked. They then set about finding a threshold below which children's haemoglobin production was not affected. The result was a threshold at about 15–18 ug/dl. This should be compared with the figure of 30 ug/dl generally said to be safe in the United States, and the then 35 ug/dl safety threshold in Britain.

The British Debate
Nowhere in the world has the issue of low level lead exposure and health been so keenly debated as in Britain. The scientific focus on the issue has been so sharp that the best understanding of the strength of the evidence of health risk can be achieved by a detailed look at the health controversy in Britain over the past few years.

In the Seventies the Conservation Society held two symposia in London. At the second, in May 1979, Needleman came from the United States to present his findings and Winneke came from Germany to review his first study and to testify that 'this pilot study has provided some evidence for an association between chronically increased childhood lead-absorption and neuropsychological impairment in children, and these results correspond very closely to those published by Needleman'. While he referred to the need to undertake further work to exclude other possible explanations, he went on 'because of the reassuring correspondence between Needleman's results and ours, however, there is more than only a chance-probability that additional research along these same lines will corroborate our findings'. (As I have already reported, his subsequent findings did corroborate the initial study.)

As a result of the growing public concern, the DHSS set up its working party under the Chairmanship of Professor Patrick Lawther. Its report has been influential since its publication in 1980, yet it is now acknowledged by some of its own members to be deeply-flawed. Lawther's terms of reference were to 'review the overall effects on health of environmental lead from all sources, and, in particular, its effects on the health and development of children, and to assess the contribution lead in petrol makes to the body burden'. (I will deal with the Lawther report's conclusions on sources of lead pollution in my next chapter, and will describe in this chapter only its findings on the health question.)

First, it noted that many uncertainties remained after its work, and it called for further research. In one sentence, for instance, it said:

> We have not been able to come to clear conclusions concerning the effects of small amounts of lead on the intelligence, behaviour and performance of children.

This should surely be read as an admission that the working party had failed to achieve its objectives and if the working party had not been able to come to any conclusions on the main question it was required to answer, it would have been far better to seek more time, or alternatively, not to publish a report at all. Instead, other contradictory passages supported a more complacent view of possible health effects, and it is these that politicians, civil servants, and the anti-knock industry seized on to substantiate their claim that there was no health hazard to children at blood lead levels below 35 ug/dl.

The Conservation Society commissioned a review of the Lawther report by Professor Derek Bryce-Smith and Dr. Robert Stephens, Reader in Chemistry at the University of Birmingham. They had in their report 'Lead or Health' two main criticisms of the Lawther report's conclusions on health:

First, it adopted an unconstructively hypercritical attitude to the studies showing effects of low levels of lead on mental functioning, but it did not subject contrary studies to the same scrutiny or scepticism.

Second, its recommendations on human over-exposure 'are unjustifiably restricted to those, including children, with blood lead levels above 35 ug/dl'. The authors stated that 'it cannot be emphasised too strongly that this figure has no real scientific or medical basis. Its adoption is likely to breed unwarranted complacency concerning the hazard to children'. As we will see later, this last sentence proved prophetic.

A particularly curious aspect of all this was the position of Professor Michael Rutter. Rutter, an internationally-respected child psychiatrist, was invited by Lawther to review the studies on low level lead exposure and health. There was an extraordinary discrepancy between Rutter's published review and the conclusions of the DHSS working party. Rutter had written of Needleman's study:

> There are a number of important questions and reservations about this study and the inferences to be drawn from it, but none of these are sufficient to invalidate the findings.

The DHSS working party, on the other hand, considering the Needleman and Winneke studies, concluded:

There are a number of reservations about these studies and the inferences to be drawn from them which in our view weaken their conclusions.

Even more curious is the contradiction between the working party's safety level of 35 ug/dl and Rutter's comment in mid-1982 that 'it never could have been justified to assume that levels below 35 ug/dl were safe'.

Rutter himself was out of the country for a considerable time during the working party's activities, and not available when the final draft was prepared. He let it be known that he would prefer not to sign it, but the DHSS and Lawther were insistent and a DHSS official travelled all the way to the US to check a draft with Rutter. Rutter now claims that the cautious conclusion was put in a context that has been 'read by many people as implying that there was positive evidence that there was an absence of effects below 35' and says:

> That would have been scientific nonsense and of course it was not the view of the working party. A paucity of evidence on ill effects (which was the case in 1980) is an entirely different matter to the presence of good evidence that there are no ill effects (which was *not* the case).

This is an extraordinary state of affairs. If Rutter's version is correct, it means that for two years a so-called safety threshold was clearly supported by the report of the working party, was adopted by Whitehall, acted upon as official policy, and at no stage did any member of the working party publicly point out to the 'many people' who had 'drawn the implication' of an absence of effects below 35, that this was 'scientific nonsense'. Nor, as the safety threshold became a matter of major scientific controversy, did anyone over two years let it be known that a threshold of 35 'was not the view of the working party'.

What possible explanation can there be for this? It is, I suppose,

---

'The only way to obtain absolute proof . . . is to expose deliberately pre-school children to different levels of lead and to then measure the resulting intellectual deficit. Clearly this proposal is ethically abhorent. . . . Children were not brought into this world to be used for experimental purposes and it is not the function of doctors to demand irrefutable evidence before taking precautionary measures. If a drug is incriminated as a cause of foetal malformation, doctors do not go on prescribing it until the case is proved beyond all doubt. The same logic applies to the use of lead in petrol and it is time that the medical profession says so in the clearest possible terms.' *World Medicine, February 20, 1982.*

---

just possible that communications were so bad, with Rutter part of the time in the US, that he was under the impression that the Committee had adopted his viewpoint when in fact it had not. This would mean the rest of the Committee were always committed to 35 ug/dl and thus have remained consistent. The other credible explanation is that the Committee did not take its responsibility for child health sufficiently seriously to correct the 'nonsense'. What I do know is that Lawther himself was more than once requested by at least one member of his working party, and also was requested by myself, to clear the matter up in 1982, and he declined to do so.

Such was the complacency the Lawther report engendered that the initial Whitehall reaction was that it should not act to reduce the official maximum of 0.40 grams per litre for lead in petrol. However, in the months between publication of the report and a Ministerial decision on this matter, Lawther was partly torpedoed by two happenings. The first, was the publication of the Yule and Lansdown pilot study. The fact that all of the children they surveyed were under the Lawther safety threshold, and that a seven point IQ deficit in children was found at half the threshold, disturbed the DHSS considerably. But what really shook Whitehall was an almost unprecedented (as he acknowledges in his opening paragraph) step by the nation's Chief Medical Officer, Sir Henry Yellowlees at the DHSS. Perturbed at the complacency and inertia, Sir Henry penned a letter to senior officials in other Ministries. (The letter was, of course, kept confidential and remained so for nearly a year until a copy was leaked to me and subsequently published in full in *The Times*.)

Sir Henry summarised the position of the Lawther Committee and the current political position, but then went on to say that:

> Further evidence has accrued which, though not in itself wholly conclusive, nevertheless strongly supports the view that . . . even at low blood levels there is a negative correlation between blood lead levels and IQ of which the simplest explanation is that the lead produces these effects.

He went on:

> There is a strong likelihood that lead in petrol is permanently reducing the IQ of many of our children. Although the reduction amounts to only a few percentage points, some hundreds of thousands of children are affected and as Chief Medical Officer I have advised my Secretary of State that action should now be taken to reduce markedly the lead content of petrol in use in the United Kingdom.
> The risk to children is now shown to be too great to take any other course. . . .

The Yellowlees letter – full text

The following is the full text of the now-famous letter written by Sir Henry Yellowlees, Chief Medical Officer at the DHSS, on March 6, 1981, and leaked to CLEAR and subsequently published in *The Times* in February 1982:

'I am taking the unusual step of writing to you about this matter which is to come before E(EA) Committee next week because the educational implications seem to me to be potentially important to DES.

It has been known for many years that lead is a hazard to health and the signs of overt lead poisoning – plumbism – are known to every medical student. More recently disquiet has grown that lead at comparatively low blood levels which are insufficient to give rise to obvious signs of lead poisoning may cause central nervous system damage to the population at large and particularly to children, with resulting minor intellectual deficits and minor behavioural disorders.

Although a good deal of environmental action has already been taken to reduce exposure to lead it was decided to set up a working party under the Chairmanship of Professor Pat Lawther to assess the situation especially with regard to children in whom low levels of exposure to lead had been detected. The Report of the Lawther Working Party was published in March 1980 and it was clear that at that time they were not convinced of the harm done by lead at low blood levels but they considered that at intermediate blood levels the risks could certainly not be discounted. Nevertheless because of the general uncertainty the Working Party recommended that the Government should take a number of measures to reduce population exposure to the metal. Further research into the problem was known to be in the pipeline and was recommended to be continued and increased.

Some of the recommendations are uncontroversial, but on one important matter – that of lead in petrol – officials from several departments involved have been unable to reach agreement and a comprehensive report will go on Monday next to E(EA) Committee of the Cabinet leaving this major item for Ministerial resolution. There is no doubt that the simplest and quickest way of reducing general population exposure to lead is by reducing sharply or by entirely eliminating lead in petrol. The Environment Departments, Health Departments and Ministry of Transport are recommending a very considerable reduction of lead in petrol, but this is opposed by the Department of Energy and the Treasury on economic grounds.

I must now make my own position clear. A year ago when the Lawther Report was published there was a degree of uncertainty, but since then further evidence has accrued which though not in itself wholly conclusive, nevertheless strongly supports the view that:

(a) Even at low blood levels there is a negative correlation between blood lead levels and IQ of which the simplest explanation is that the lead produces these effects.

(b) Lead in petrol is a major contributor to blood lead acting through the food-chain as well as by inhalation.

Further research is being mounted but we are dealing here with the biological sciences where truly conclusive evidence may be unobtainable

The combination of widespread criticism of the Lawther report, and publication of the subsequent Yule and Lansdown pilot study and the Yellowlees letter, opened up a substantial debate, and, as we shall see later, this forced Ministers' hands, and a reduction of lead in petrol (but not unfortunately, its elimination) was decided upon.

CLEAR decided in 1982 to put the medical and scientific evidence on the line. It invited the authors of all the main studies to an international symposium in London to present and update their work and submit it to cross-examination. CLEAR went out of its way to offer every known critic of these researchers the opportunity to cross-examine or contradict the evidence. It invited all the relevant Ministries, every member of the Lawther Committee, all the industrial companies concerned with lead in petrol, and also advertised the symposium widely within the medical and scientific world, to environmental health officers and others. No-one (apart, inevitably, from Associated Octel) subsequently questioned the scientific integrity of the event. Key to its importance, however, would be the choice of Chairman. We decided to invite Professor Michael Rutter. Rutter had in fact till then avoided the lead debate

---

and it is therefore doubtful whether there is anything to be gained by deferring a decision until the results of further research become available.

There is a strong likelihood that lead in petrol is permanently reducing the IQ of many of our children. Although the reduction amounts to only a few percentage points, some hundreds of thousands of children are affected and as Chief Medical Officer I have advised my Secretary of State that action should now be taken to reduce markedly the lead content of petrol in use in the United Kingdom.

The risk to children is now shown to be too great for me to take any other course and I am therefore conveying this advice to you as Permanent Secretary in DES and I am copying the letter to the Permanent Secretaries at the Home Office and the Department of the Environment being the other Government Departments to which I owe responsibility.

You will know that several other major industrial nations faced with similar problems have opted for lead-free petrol or for petrol with a very low lead level despite the substantial cost and the energy penalties so incurred.

I regard this as a very serious issue on which I should give you my opinion as Chief Medical Officer.' Sir Henry Yellowlees, Chief Medical Officer.

Sir Henry then added in a footnote:

'The health evidence, persuasive though it is already, cannot yet be described as conclusive. The important thing is that new evidence is accumulating all the time – and it always points in the same direction as the existing evidence, so that the health case becomes steadily stronger and stronger.'

since the publication of the Lawther report, and on the available evidence we had to assume that he remained loyal to the position of the Lawther Committee. There were, however, two reasons for our choice: first, of all those involved in the lead controversy, Rutter was the one man whom we knew people on all sides of the debate respected as a man of exceptional scientific reputation and independence of mind. Second, we knew we had to take the risk of inviting a Chairman who could not possibly be assumed to be sympathetic towards, let alone supportive of, CLEAR. Furthermore, he was a man who could not, should he conclude that the evidence supported our case, be brushed aside by Ministers or civil servants, let alone fellow scientists.

On the final day of the symposium Rutter summarised his view of the evidence (my quotations are from the revised version of his speech prepared for the published proceedings):

Of the pre-1980 research he said: 'The great majority (but not quite all) investigations have found slight but significant differences between the intelligence and behaviour of children with high lead levels compared with those of children with low lead levels. . . . These findings are not in any reasonable doubt but there has been much dispute on the interpretation to be placed on them. Three issues have dominated that debate: first, the uncertainty as to whether the statistical associations reflect the causal effect . . . ; secondly, the uncertainty on the level of lead exposure at which such effects may occur; and thirdly, doubts on the reliability and validity of both the measures of body lead burden and measures of neuropsychological impairment.'

He then reviewed the more recent evidence from Needleman, Winneke, and Yule and Lansdown, as well as other studies, and concluded: 'In summary, the new evidence since 1980 has been consistent in pointing to significant effects at the low levels of lead exposure (below 40 ug/dl) where there was most doubt on the basis of the earlier studies. Also, the recent investigations have been able to demonstrate that the effects tend to be maintained (although substantially reduced) after control for possible confounding variables. However, in addition, they have confirmed earlier findings in their indication that the effects on psychological functioning tend to be relatively small'.

Discussing the quality of the available measures of both the body lead burden and of neuropsychological function, he emphasised that the main doubt had been concerned with the amount of random error in these measures, rather than the presence of systematic bias. 'Accordingly, in so far as errors have been present, they will have tended to result in an *under*- rather than an over-estimate of the effects of lead.'

He then drew on a widely-accepted list of requirements for inferring a cause and effect relationship from the data.

Firstly, there was the question of the consistency of the observed association – had it been repeatedly noted in different investigations using different research strategies? The short answer on that point was 'Yes, the observed associations have been reasonably consistent', and this lent some support to the causal inference.

> Secondly, there is the matter of a biological gradient, or dose-response curve. In other words, if there were a causal relationship it would be expected that low levels of lead would have minor effects, moderate levels of lead should have rather greater effects, and high levels of lead should have the greatest effect of all . . . this is a particularly important point, as the failure to find a dose-response relationship undoubtedly would cast serious doubt on the causal hypothesis.

He said there was some evidence of a dose-response relationship within most studies, but a lack of consistency with respect to the biological gradient if results were compared *across* studies. However, he said, he was less inclined to place weight on the lack of a dose-response relationship across studies than he had been in the past: firstly, because comparisons across studies do not necessarily involve the same standard; secondly, because of the numerous other powerful influences involved with intelligence and behaviour, and the likelihood of those variances to vary from sample to sample, so that the effects of lead at different doses could not be compared meaningfully; and thirdly, because there is not a very close degree of comparability between different approaches to the measurement of lead. Until ways can be quickly found around these faults, 'we are forced to rely on the regularity of dose-response relationships *within* studies. Those data are sparse, but, on the whole, they are consistent with the causal argument'.

Moving on down his list of requirements for inferring a cause and effect relationship, he came to:

> the last two considerations that stem from (the) list of requirements for cause and effect relationships. These concern the strength and specificity of the association. There is no doubt, that causal inferences are much more likely to be correct when the associations are both strong and specific. Thus, the hypothesis that cigarette smoking predisposes to cancer of the lung is powerfully supported by the fact that the association is a strong one and by the fact that the association is specifically with cancer of the lung and not with cancer generally. When associations are weak and general there must always be doubt

about the causal hypothesis. Perhaps, it is this fact more than any other that has made many people sceptical about the reality of the supposed psychological sequelae to low level lead exposure. Does the generality of the suggested effects of lead toxicity cast doubt on the causal hypothesis? It does not. The point is that the evidence with respect to other forms of trauma to the brain are reasonably consistent in showing that the effects tend to impair a wide range of brain systems rather than just one. We may conclude that, far from throwing doubt on the causal hypothesis, the generality of effects is entirely consistent with what might have been anticipated from what is known concerning brain function and malfunction.

What, then, about the weakness of association?

To begin with, we do need to be quite clear that the association is indeed a weak one. All, but all, of the studies are consistent in showing that low level lead exposure is associated with deficits in the order of three to five points of IQ and with moderate increases in the proportion of children showing attentional deficits or hyperactivity . . . but to what extent does the weakness of the association throw doubts on the causal hypothesis? Perhaps the most crucial point is that there is no way strong associations could be found. This is because we know there are many powerful genetic and environmental influences on intelligence and behaviour. Lead could *add* to these but it could not be expected to replace them. Accordingly, weak associations are not necessarily inconsistent with the causal hypothesis. On the contrary, they are to be expected.

He considered once more the possibility that the association between lead and psychological impairment could be due to some other uncontrolled social variable and acknowledged this was a possibility:

But, even on the evidence available to us now, it would not seem likely that social variables will explain away the whole of the apparent effects of lead on psychological functioning. This is because in the studies undertaken so far, many of the effects of lead have remained even after the introduction of statistical controls for appropriate social variables and because the associations hold in the investigations with the greatest social controls. We cannot be sure that the effects of lead are real but the balance of evidence suggests they are.

He concluded this section of his speech with a reminder of the proposal by philosopher Sir Karl Popper that the way of science did not consist in any proof of a hypothesis; rather, it consisted of a series of failures to disprove the hypothesis.

By this standard, it is evident that the best of the most recent studies have indeed failed to disprove the hypothesis that low level lead exposure leads to psychological impairment. Inevitably, for the reasons that I have discussed at some length, there are doubts, but, as a result of the further research that has been conducted over the past few years, these doubts are less than they were some time ago. The implication is that it would be both safer in practice, and scientifically more appropriate, to act as if the hypothesis were true rather than to do nothing on the assumption that it might be false.

Rutter then went on to demolish the safety threshold of 35 ug/dl, stating that all of the studies that had examined effects in the range below 35 ug/dl –

have demonstrated effects and none has produced evidence that there is a threshold below which there is safety. Of course, it is likely that effects are less frequent and less severe at lower levels of lead exposure, and it may be that there is a point at which ill effects are so extremely rare that they can be discounted for all practical purposes. However, *if there is such a threshold it has yet to be determined*. At present, all that one can conclude is that it now seems much more likely than hitherto that there are effects at levels below 35 ug/dl and that we cannot specify any range of safety. The animal evidence points to the same conclusion.

Winding up, Professor Rutter said:

the research findings tell us that there is a probability (although not certainty) that low level lead exposure may have important adverse psychological effects. These effects are not large and it is clear that there are many other more important influences on psychological function. Moreover, it is probable that there are considerable individual differences to susceptibility . . . but, the risk seems to be substantially more than a trivial one and, at least in some individuals, the effects are likely to be of practical importance in causing impairment of functioning. The implication is that we now know enough to warrant taking such public health actions as are likely to reduce lead pollution in the environment, provided such actions do not have other hazards, and provided they are not prohibitively expensive. . . . The removal of lead from petrol would seem to be one of those worthwhile and safe public health actions. The evidence suggests that the removal of lead from petrol would have a quite substantial effect in reducing lead pollution and the costs are quite modest by any reasonable standard. . . . In my view, the reduction of lead in petrol to an intermediate level is an unacceptable compromise without clear advantages and with definite disadvantages.

Why was the reduction to 0.15 grams per litre inadequate? Because there was no evidence of a safety threshold for blood lead levels. There was considerable individual variation in susceptibility to lead – a variation that applies to most toxins.

One person's safety limit is in someone else's danger zone. It is for that reason that in establishing the safety limit for the dosage of drugs, the limit is set well below that at which ill effects generally appear.

There were, too, geographical variations. He went on:

> It is for those reasons that we have to set a limit for lead well below that at which adverse effects commonly appear. Unless there is a very substantial gap between the overall population limit and the usual threshold (if there is one) of toxicity, some individuals will suffer. The cost of setting the safety limit too high, therefore, is that some children will be damaged unnecessarily.
>
> The reduction of lead would not bring about *major* improvements in the health of British children as a whole and we should not create false expectations. But the reduction of lead in the environment should make some worthwhile difference to some children and that ought to constitute a quite sufficient justification for action now.

So there it was. And there it is.

All of those who had campaigned to establish that children were *at risk* of harm because of lead exposure at much lower levels than previously acknowledged – at *normal* levels of exposure – no longer stood alone. As this objective professor of international distinction had demonstrated, the best scientific and medical evidence available supported CLEAR's view.

Even as he spoke a document was on its way to the Royal Commission on Environmental Pollution from the British Medical Association. It was to add further to the trend of opinion. On the safety threshold, it said:

> For operational and regulatory purposes it would be desirable to set levels for zones considered dangerous, unacceptable, acceptable or safe, but there is little justification for such classification on biological or toxicological grounds. It is probable that there is a continuum of harm, and there may well be levels at which the risk is negligible. However, there is a high degree of individual susceptibility to damage from lead.

Of the safety level of 35 ug/dl, the BMA said:

> There is evidence that children who have body burdens of lead lower than that indicated by 30 ug/dl may be at risk. Associations have been demonstrated between impairment of mental functioning and lead levels below the range previously considered harmful. At first there was some doubt about the validity of these studies but it is now generally accepted that the association is real and it should not therefore be disregarded. . . . On the basis of the evidence which it has received the BMA considers that lead is capable of causing harm at levels of

exposure previously considered safe, i.e. at levels indicated by lead between 30 ug/dl–80 ug/dl. It therefore recommends that steps should be taken to reduce lead in the environment by progressive measures so as to protect those at risk.

The Key Word is RISK

Throughout this chapter I have placed much emphasis on the word *risk*. Some politicians and bureaucrats, and even some medics and scientists, insist on 'conclusive' evidence of harm. But, what is conclusive? As Dr. Needleman has observed, the issue of lead and health involves 'complex issues encompassing data from many disciplines including chemistry, pharmacology, neurobiology, psychology, epidemiology'. The scientific debate on the issue has clearly demonstrated that what is 'conclusive' to one scientist is inconclusive to another, and it could take years to reconcile the differences.

Some of the most reputable scientists say that it may never be possible to achieve conclusive evidence of harm to children from low level lead exposure.

Sir Henry Yellowlees, Chief Medical Officer at the DHSS, has said:

> Further research is being mounted, but we are dealing here with the biological sciences where truly conclusive evidence may be unattainable and it is therefore doubtful whether there is anything to be gained by deferring a decision until the results of further research become available.

Professor Philip Graham, a London Child Psychiatrist involved in Medical Research Council-sponsored work on lead and health, has written:

> It may be the issues will remain unresolved, even after further research has been carried out.

Professor Rutter has said:

> There are inevitable doubts and uncertainties surrounding the findings of all the empirical investigations. It is important to realise, of course, that this is not an unusual state of affairs in science. Studies in the real world have to deal with complex situations and with many influences of different kinds that are difficult to disentangle. No one study ever finally resolves the scientific questions in these circumstances and it would be scientifically foolish as well as politically irresponsible to wait for the perfect study to be undertaken.

In the famous 1975–76 case before the United States Court of Appeals when the anti-knock industry tried to have the American controls on lead in petrol over-turned, the court confronted this very issue. In its judgement it pointed out that the Administrator of the Environment Protection Agency had interpreted his responsibility to deal with lead emissions from cars 'that will endanger the public health or welfare' or such emissions as 'present a significant *risk* of harm to the health of urban populations, particularly to the health of city children'. The anti-knock industry claimed that the Administrator had erroneously interpreted the Clean Air Act by not sufficiently appreciating the rigour demanded by the 'will endanger' standard. In the court's own words:

> Petitioners (i.e. the industries) argued that the 'will endanger' standard requires a high quantum of factual proof, proof of actual harm rather than of a 'significant risk of harm' . . . since, according to petitioners, regulations must be premised upon actual proof of actual harm, the Administrator has, in their view, no power to assess risks or make policy judgements in deciding to regulate lead additives.

The court concluded: *'We have considered these arguments with care and find them to be without merit.'* It continued:

> Case law and dictionary definitions are in accord that endanger means something *less than actual harm*. When one is endangered, harm is *threatened*; no actual injury need ever occur. Thus, a town may be 'endangered' by a threatened plague or hurricane and yet emerge from the danger completely unscathed. A statute allowing for regulation in the face of danger is, necessarily, a precautionary statute. Regulatory action may be taken before the threatened harm occurs; indeed, the very existence of such precautionary legislation would seem to *demand* that regulatory action proceed, and, optimally, prevent the perceived threat.

The circuit judge of the Court of Appeals, J. Skelly Wright, said:

> the statutes, and common sense, demand regulatory action to prevent harm, even if the regulator is less than certain that harm is otherwise inevitable.

Those concerned with lead pollution who argue from this position will stress that any responsible doctor should, when taking medical decisions, err on the side of prudence. If that is the policy for the individual patient, so it should be the policy when it comes to public health. In their view we should act on the basis of risk because the other option is to demand of one generation of children after another that they should be used for experimental purposes. We then, of course, find ourselves involved in a discussion about levels of risk. There are three factors we must consider:

(1) *the nature of the risk to the individual.*

We have already established that at risk is the mental health of children. Thus, the risk, if established, *is* of a serious nature.

(2) *the number of individuals at risk.*

As we shall see in the next chapter, a vast number of children are exposed; at the very minimum, every child in urban circumstances is at risk in Britain. Thus, the scale of risk in terms of potential victims is considerable.

(3) *the practicality of individuals acting themselves to avoid the risk.*

There is no way whereby the individual can avoid the risk involved. This differentiates this debate from, say, the control of cigarettes, where there is a voluntary aspect. On the whole it is the cigarette smoker who is most likely to be adversely affected by the practice and he or she has taken a voluntary decision after considerable public education on the risks involved, and can legitimately claim that regulation of his or her cigarette smoking would be an infringement of individual freedom. However, the individual takes no decision to be exposed to lead pollution from car exhausts.

The answer to those three points, then, is that:

(1) the risk is of a serious nature,
(2) a vast number of children are at risk, and
(3) the risk is unavoidable, except by a central communal decision to eliminate sources of lead pollution.

This is indeed a high level of risk.

There are many others, however, who will argue that we are beyond the evidence of risk. Their view is well represented by my colleague in CLEAR, Dr. Robin Russell Jones:

> If you have a scientific thesis, namely that there is a causal association between lead and reduced intelligence, then you have to construct a

---

'Uncertainties in scientific knowledge have limited the ability to establish definitive, quantitive relationships between levels of lead in the environment and risks of adverse effects on human health. . . . Government agencies therefore have had to make arbitrary scientific judgements, as well as social, subjective decisions about how much risk and how much uncertainty are acceptable. Recent actions by Congress and the Courts reflect the consensus that it is better to proceed with decisions in the face of uncertainty than to risk the consequences of inaction.' *Lead in the Human Environment*, US *National Academy of Science report.*

---

series of studies to test that thesis and attempt to find some other explanation for the association. No matter how many times you demonstrate an association you will not have provided conclusive proof, but equally the failure to disprove the association strengthens the basic thesis. So the situation with lead is as follows: all of the most recent and all of the best-designed studies have indeed shown an association between lead and mental impairment. The question that arises is how many more studies are necessary before the thesis becomes so strongly supported that action is necessary. As far as risk is concerned, the risk was of course there before the association was established and in 1973 the United States was prepared to take a decision on the basis of that risk. What in Britain we are asking the authorities to do is to act not on the basis of risk but on the basis of a thesis being reinforced every time a new set of results is published. If we want to talk about risk, then we have to say that the first risk taken was to put lead in petrol. When it was demonstrated in the Sixties that this had caused environmental contamination on a global scale we took an even bigger risk by allowing the practice to continue. When preliminary observations from the United States in the early Seventies showed associations between low level lead exposure and mental impairment many people, including the Americans, found the risk unacceptable. With the publication of the Needleman and Winneke studies, the proposition that lead affects intelligence in children extended beyond risk and became the best explanation for the available data. The risk at that point became intolerable. Subsequent research has reinforced those studies. It is at this point that many serious scientists now feel able to belatedly commit themselves.

Whether the evidence I have described is of serious risk to public health, or of discernable damage, I believe it justifies all reasonable action. In the next chapter I hope to demonstrate that the priority has to be a ban on lead in petrol.

3.
The invisible cloud

'Now, I don't want to be an alarmist! I do not suggest that people die in the streets from automobile exhaust. But over the past quarter century more and more data have been developed that suggest that the exhaust from motor vehicles contributes to degraded health of urban populations.' *Eric O. Stork, from 1970–78 Deputy Assistant Administrator of the US Environmental Protection Agency, responsible for the USA Automobile Emission Control Programme.*

LEAD IS a metal abundantly available in the earth's crust, easy to mine and to smelt from the ore. It has a low melting point, is soft, malleable, ductile, and does not corrode easily. Because of these qualities it was one of the first metals to be widely used by man and is now produced in far greater quantities than any other toxic heavy metal. Across the world about 3.5 million tonnes are produced every year. While it is mined in over 40 countries, four of these, the USSR, the USA, Australia and Canada, produce 60%.

The toxic effects of lead have been known since the second century BC. This did not stop its widespread use by the Greeks and the Romans, who made water pipes from lead, and also containers for wine and other drinks. For some reason man has always been particularly stubborn in his refusal to respond to the dangers posed by lead. Indeed, Benjamin Franklin once commented on this – 'How long a useful truth may be known and exist, before it is generally received and practised on'. The increased use of lead during the industrial revolution produced several forms of occupational lead poisoning, not least in women. There were reports of sterility, abortion, stillbirth and premature delivery (indeed, lead was once used as an aid to abortion). This led to controls on the employment of women in lead industries.

Jane S. Lin-Fu records in a 1980 book on lead effects edited by Needleman the growth of evidence of lead poisoning in the United States in this century caused by pica (persistent eating of leaded paint), proximity to various industrial uses, the burning by poverty-stricken families of discarded storage battery casings for fuel in cold weather, and lead in cans of food. Between 1950 and 1960 there were 611 cases of lead poisoning and 48 deaths in the city of Baltimore alone. In New York between 1950 and 1954 there were

143 cases with 39 deaths, and in Philadelphia between 1955 and 1960 there were 223 cases with 41 fatalities. Between 1959 and 1961 there were 429 cases and 67 deaths in Chicago. In the mid-Sixties, Lin-Fu reports. . .

> came the discovery that lead poisoning, a preventable illness, was occuring in epidemic proportions in many inner city slums. . . . Moreover, excessive exposure to lead was more widespread than had been presumed, . . . the problem was not confined to the poor or to the eastern part of the country; it was in fact a nationwide phenomenon. These findings . . . finally led to acknowledgement in the late 1960's that lead poisoning was an important public health pediatric problem.

Over the years regulations on exposure to lead were tightened and in Britain, as in the United States, cases of classical lead poisoning have been substantially reduced by governmental intervention, and also by tighter safety measures within the affected industries.

Unfortunately, as can be demonstrated from the behaviour of many other industries, danger to public health is to many companies an irritating obstacle to be overcome, a public relations problem, rather than a reason to seek profits elsewhere. There is no record of any company concerned with the production and sale of lead acknowledging that their product is a threat to the health of the population as a whole, just as there is no record of any petroleum company, or any company connected with the anti-knock industry, making such a concession.

The lead and anti-knock industries have based their defence on two arguments:

First, they claim that a significant proportion of lead is natural and that we are exposed to it simply because it is there – in the earth's crust. They suggest that the lead we absorb from food comes naturally from the soil into the roots of plants.

Second, each industry seeks to lay the blame for industrial lead pollution on another. Thus the paint industry blames the anti-knock industry and vice versa.

In this chapter, therefore, I will deal with those claims.

It is Not Natural; We Poison Ourselves

The best way to establish where responsibility lies for the earth's increasing contamination by lead is to compare lead levels today with lead levels before man began to mine and use it. This may sound impossible, but in fact the information exists and measurements can be made.

A number of scientists have contributed to our knowledge in this area but the key researcher has been Clair Patterson, now 60, a geochemist at the California Institute of Technology, who for nearly 20 years has been studying the build-up of lead in the earth and in the air. As the US magazine *Environmental Science and Technology* said in 1981:

> The debate over the extent of contamination of the contemporary environment has been all but put to rest by Patterson's work. He has shown contamination of the oceans of the northern hemisphere 10-fold over prehistoric levels; the atmosphere, 50 fold; the Greenland ice-cap, 300-fold; and most American bodies 500-fold. Most significantly, he has demonstrated that conflicting results obtained by others were the result of contamination of samples and laboratory equipment, leading to analytical errors of as much as three orders of magnitude in the numbers they obtain for prehistoric levels.

The magazine describes why Patterson's results are more reliable than that of other scientists:

> He takes elaborate precautions to prevent contamination of his samples in his laboratory by the elevated levels of lead that are omnipresent in the modern environment. The interior of his laboratory is lined with plastic; an air-lock and pressurised ultraclean air prevent outside contaminated air from entering and his reagents are cleaned of lead contamination within the lab. His precautions – and his use of the most sensitive analytic technique for lead, isotope dilution mass spectrometry – have given him the edge needed to detect the true, minute quantities of lead occuring in samples that reflect the prehistoric environment. And he has shown time and time again that conflicting results obtained by other workers are the result of sample contamination and inadequate analytic techniques.

By the analysis of prehistoric skeletal remains in ultraclean laboratory conditions, Patterson has been able to demonstrate that we in our industrialised society have in our bodies 500 times the lead content of pre-industrial prehistoric man. Patterson illustrates the level of contamination with figure 4. He represents the lead content in bodies in dots, with one dot to represent natural levels as found in

---

'The levels of lead in present-day Americans probably are two to three orders of magnitude higher than natural levels of lead in humans.' (This means 100–1,000 times greater.) *Lead in the Human Environment*, National Academy of Sciences report, USA, 1980.

---

prehistoric man, 2,000 dots to represent a man with 'classical lead poisoning', and 500 dots to represent you and I. We already have a lead level 500 times prehistoric predecessors and a quarter of the way to classical lead poisoning.

Patterson has also measured the increase in another way, at the same time establishing the worldwide extent of industrial lead pollution. For instance, he took measurements from snow strata in the northern ice-cap dating back to 1800 BC. He found a 300-fold increase in the lead levels with most of the increase occurring in the past fifty years. Since these huge fluctuations cannot be accounted for in terms of natural lead, it must follow that the much heavier lead content nearer the surface reflects the widespread dispersal of industrial lead to remote corners of the globe. (As no-one has been using paint in the area, nor are there water pipes, the contamination is obviously caused by airborne lead and no-one denies that at least 90% of all airborne lead comes from car exhausts.)

Patterson's work and conclusions first became widely known as a result of an article in the *US Archives of Environmental Health* in

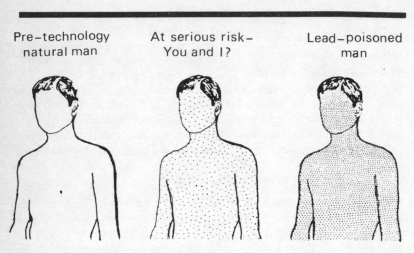

Pre-technology natural man   At serious risk– You and I?   Lead-poisoned man

Figure 4   COMPARISON OF relative amounts of lead in people: natural amount found in prehistoric people on the left; average amount found in present-day Americans in the middle with subtle effects on mental function already likely, especially in children; and minimum amount which will cause classical lead poisoning in a significant fraction of a group of people on the right. Each dot represents a unit of lead equivalent to $3 \times 10^{1}/_4 gPb/70$ kg person, based on a prehistoric natural skeletal value Pb/Ca (atomic) $= 6 \times 10^{1}/_8$ at age 45. Source: Dr. Clair Patterson, CLEAR Symposium, 1982

1965. He concluded a lengthy summary of his research and findings with these words:

> There are definite indications that residents of the United States today are undergoing severe chronic lead insult. The average American ingests some 400 ug of lead per day in food, air and water, a process which has been viewed with complacency for decades. Geochemical relationships and material balance considerations show that this ingestion of about 20 tonnes of lead per year on a national basis is grossly excessive compared with natural conditions. . . . Existing rates of lead absorption are about 30 times higher than inferred natural rates, yielding body burdens (and blood concentrations) of values about 100 times above inferred natural levels. . . . It appears that the following activities deserve serious consideration and support: defining natural and toxic levels with greater care than in the past; investigating deleterious effects of severe chronic lead insult; investigating the dispersion of industrial lead in the food chain; elimination of some of the most serious sources of lead pollution, such as lead alkyl (lead in petrol), insecticides, food-can solder, water service pipes, kitchenware glazes, paint; and a re-evaluation by persons in positions of responsibility in the field of public health of their role in this matter.

The paper aroused considerable concern, not least within the lead and anti-knock industry. Patterson lost some sources of research finance and was brutally criticised. However, over the years his opposition, mostly industrial scientists, have failed to effectively challenge him, and the magazine *Environmental Science and Technology* concluded in 1981 that in the face of his '. . . overwhelming body of evidence, resistance to Patterson's findings can be attributed largely to politics and professional pride – no-one likes to be told that his analytic technique is off by a factor of 1,000!'

The scientific evidence of a vast increase in lead pollution as a result of its industrial use is not limited to Patterson's work alone. More recently, scientists from other countries have also pursued research in this area and produced similar findings.

It is, I suppose, necessary that scientists should sometimes devote years of research to demonstrate the obvious, but I cannot resist suggesting that it really is plain common sense, downright obvious, that if man was not mining and using lead at all a few centuries back and is now mining and using 3.5 million tonnes of lead a year – lead that is withdrawn from under the earth's crust and circulated and widely dispersed – we *must* be more efficiently exposed to much more lead than our predecessors. Thus, when industrialists say that most of our lead exposure comes from natural sources in the soil, they not only over-ride the scientific facts, but stretch to the extreme the boundaries of common sense and credibility.

What we, in fact, know is that after 50 years of using lead in petrol, it is present in our lives every hour of every day – we breathe it, we eat and drink it, and we have it at unacceptable levels in our bodies. The US National Academy of Science said in 1980:

> The environment of the United States is pervasively contaminated with lead . . . every member of the population of the United States is exposed to elevated levels of lead in air, drinking water, and foods – levels that are present because of human activities.

But is the Problem Lead in Petrol?

When confronted with the weakness of their claim that lead pollution is from natural sources, the defenders of lead in petrol switch to their second line of defence – that airborne lead (or lead from petrol) is a minor contributor to body lead burdens.

Their case can be summed up like this:

> *'The use of lead in petrol adds 10% to human intake. After emission from car exhausts, it becomes airborne lead. Much of that simply disappears into space. The real problem is lead in food (some of it derived naturally from the soil and some from processing and canning procedures), lead in paint, especially in urban areas where there are a lot of older houses, lead from localised sources, such as smelters or factories using it, lead in water pipes and whatever. Lead pollution is a multi-source problem and it makes no sense to persecute the anti-knock industry when it represents such a small source of pollution and saves money and energy.'*

It is, indeed, the case that lead is a major, multi-source, neurotoxic environmental pollutant, and that the only prudent public health course is to reduce or eliminate *every* source of exposure. One cannot over-state the danger to some Scottish children from old water pipes and the need to eliminate them, or the threat to

---

'The legitimate causes for concern over the possible health hazards of current levels of lead in the atmosphere are both very real and clearly supported by scientific evidence. . . . Our panel report clearly points out that infants and young people and possibly some workers exposed to dense vehicular traffic are subject to hazard.' *Dr. Paul Hammond, member of the Atmospheric Lead Study Panel of the National Academy of Science, USA, in 'Saturday Review', 1971.*

---

children still exposed to old heavily-leaded paint, or the need, particularly in Britain, where industry is controlled more by voluntary understandings than by firm regulations, for decisive measures to eliminate lead from food containers, toys, and any other products they come into contact with. It is also a fact that most cases of clinical lead poisoning are caused by intensive exposure to localised sources of these sorts. However, for most people lead in petrol is their major source of lead. It is responsible for at least one third and probably two thirds of human lead intake and a ban on lead in petrol represents the quickest, most effective, and least expensive way of reducing lead levels in the population as a whole. While *some* children in *some* areas may be more dangerously exposed to a particular localised source demanding local protest and local action, they, as well as the population as a whole, will benefit from the reduced lead intake from petrol. As the Center for Disease Control in the United States commented:

> The reduction in mean blood lead levels (as a result of reductions in lead in petrol) does mean that the high-risk young children living near to high-dose sources of lead (i.e. leaded paint, lead already deposited in dust and soil, etc) will have a greater margin of safety.

Lead in petrol contributes at least 90% of lead to air because most of the industrial lead processes produce large lead particles which 'fall out' close to the source, while the internal combustion engine is so designed that it produces a fine aerosol of infinitesimally small particles. These remain airborne for longer, travel huge distances with the prevailing winds, and are ultimately readily inhaled and absorbed into the body. Thus the addition of lead to petrol has, in the words of Russell Jones and Stephens, 'created a source of lead unique in terms of its capacity to pollute on a global scale and in terms of its ability to gain access to the human system'.

The tragedy is that many of the causes of classical lead poisoning were at last being effectively confronted in the 1920's just at the time industrial chemists in the United States were making the discovery that was to create a far greater hazard for a far greater number of people all over the world. It was T. Midgley, Jr, with C. F. Kettering, T. A. Boyd, and co-workers in the research laboratories of General Motors who invented the anti-knock compounds or lead alkyls known as tetraethyl lead (TEL) and tetramethyl lead (TML) to prevent engine 'knock' or 'pinking'.

The petroleum industry wasted no time in capitalising on the invention. In less than a year the Ethyl Corporation and Du Ponts were manufacturing the additive, and on February 2, 1923, the first leaded petrol (or gasoline as it is known in the United States) was sold. Unfortunately, some manufacturers had not taken adequate safety measures for their employees and more than 100 became seriously ill or insane and a number of people died.

Known deaths included:

Sept. 21, 1923, one death, E I du Pont de Nemours & Co., Carney's Point, NJ.

June 1, 1924, two deaths, General Motors Research Corporation, Dayton, Ohio.

July 14, 1924, one death, E I du Pont de Nemours & Co., Carney's Point, NJ.

Oct. 20, 1924, one death, E I du Pont de Nemours & Co., Carney's Point, NJ.

Oct. 28–30, 1924, five deaths, Standard Oil Company, Bayway, NJ.

Feb. 18, 1925, one death, E I du Pont de Nemours & Co., Carney's Point, NJ.

Feb. 18, 1925, one insane, Standard Oil Company, Bayway, NJ.

Symptoms were described as:

A marked fall in blood pressure, sometimes 60mm of mercury below normal, an accompanying fall in body temperature, which has been as low as 94.6F, and a low pulse rate, down to 48 a minute. Then symptoms of profound cerebral involvement appear, persistent insomnia, extraordinary restlessness and talkativeness, and delusions. The gait is like that of a drunken man, but there are no paralyses or convulsions. Finally, after a period of exaggerated movements of all of the muscles of the body, with sweating, the patient becomes violently manical, shouting, leaping from the bed, smashing furniture, and acting as if in delirium tremens; morphine only accentuates the symptoms. The patient may finally die in exhaustion. In two fatal cases, the body temperature rose to 110F just before death occurred. One of these was a young man of fine physique who had been at work only five weeks. He is said to have suffered terrible agony. 'He died yelling'.

As a result, the manufacture and distribution was stopped in May, 1925, while the public health authorities and the industries concerned worked out safety regulations for the production of the additive, for its mixture with petrol, and for its distribution and sale.

Incidentally, during the Second World War there were reports of 25 cases of poisoning by tetraethyl lead in Britain, two of them fatal, as a result of men cleaning storage tanks for leaded petrol. War conditions in countries of the Middle East and Far East made the cleaning of tanks difficult to supervise 'and there were 200 cases of poisoning with 40 deaths'. In 1947 two Italians died after using leaded petrol for the dry cleaning of clothes. In 1968 *The Times* reported that a Greek court had sentenced three executives of a rubber shoe factory to prison after the deaths since 1964 of four workers and the insanity of 11 others as a result of tetraethyl lead poisoning. Scientists testified the disease was due to poisoning by 'tetraethyl lead contained in cheap petrol used in the factories'.

Three major studies have over the past few years served to incriminate leaded petrol as a significant source of lead exposure.

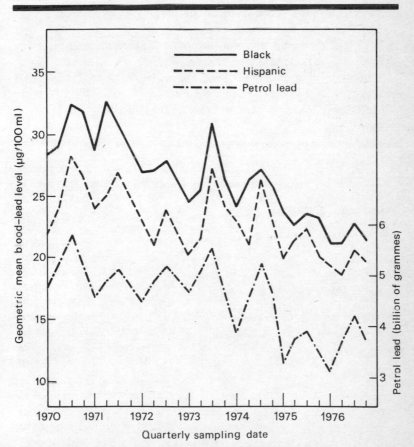

Figure 5 RELATIONSHIPS BETWEEN sales of petrol-lead in New York area and blood-lead levels of New York children (n = 178,533). Blood-lead levels of white children were similar to those of Hispanic children (largely Puerto Ricans). From a Report by I. H. Billick et al., Department of Housing and Urban Development, Washington DC, USA, 1979.

The first was undertaken by Dr. Irwin Billick, a senior US Government researcher. He first monitored the blood lead levels of over 178,000 children in the New York area and compared them with the sales of leaded petrol in the same area. Figure 5 shows what an impressive association he was able to demonstrate between the two. He then went on to compare the geometric mean blood lead levels and the amount of lead in petrol used in a three-state area surrounding New York city and once more demonstrated an extra-ordinary correlation between the two. On the whole, he found that blood-lead correlated more closely with petrol-lead than with air-lead and attributed this to a substantial input from petrol-lead via other pathways than direct inhalation.

Even more formidable evidence from the United States has been provided by a huge survey into trends in blood lead levels in the United States population between 1976 and 1980, known as the Health and Nutrition Examination Survey (NHANES). This involved a sample of 27,801 persons aged 6 months to 74 years from 64 areas of the United States between the years 1976 and 1980 – the first four

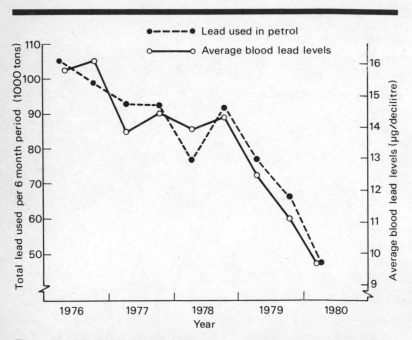

Figure 6   LEAD USED in gasoline production and blood-lead levels, February 1976– February 1980. Source: NHANES data presented by Dr. Lee Annest to CLEAR Symposium 1982.

years of the programme to phase lead out of petrol. In that time lead in petrol in the United States was reduced by 55 per cent and there was a corresponding 36.7% decline in blood lead levels. Decreases were found in all races, ages, and both sexes. Further analysis indicated that the reduction was not due to seasonal sampling, income sampling, geographic region sampling, urban versus rural sampling, laboratory measurement error, or chance (see figures 6 and 7). While Dr. Lee Annest of the National Center for Health Statistics, who presented the results of the survey to the CLEAR symposium in London in May 1982, is a statistician and did not seek to interpret the data in any depth, he concluded:

> The striking similarity between the decrease in the use of lead in the production of petrol and the drop in mean NHANES blood lead levels indicates that lead entering the atmosphere from the combustion of leaded petrol contributes significantly to the level of lead in human blood.

A number of anti-lead measures were taken in the United States during this time, and it is fair to assume that a proportion of the fall in blood lead levels is due to them; but the dramatic fall at the same time as there was an equally dramatic fall in the use of lead in petrol does, in the words of Dr. Vernon Houk, Acting Director of the US Center for Environmental Health's Center for Disease Control, 'clearly demonstrate that as we have removed lead from

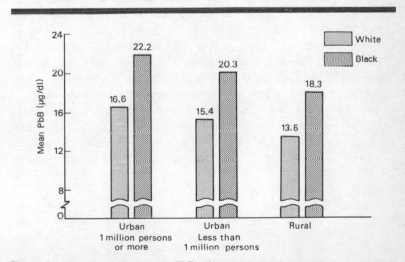

Figure 7 MEAN BLOOD lead levels (PbB) of children ages six months to five years by degree of urbanization: United States, 1976–80. Source: National Health and Nutrition Examination Survey, National Center for Health Statistics

petrol we have also removed lead from ourselves and our children'.

In 1982 the Environmental Protection Agency in the United States arranged for sophisticated statistical techniques to be applied to a combination of the NHANES study, the Billick study, and some others. Crucial conclusions were:

1   The restrictions imposed by EPA on the use of lead in petrol refining in recent years has significantly reduced the average amount of lead in blood.
2   During the period 1976 through 1980 an estimated 46% of the blood lead of the average American was due to petrol lead emissions.
3   Black children have higher blood lead levels than older blacks or whites as a result of exposure to the same levels of petrol lead emissions. During the same 1976 to 1980 period, an estimated 62% of their blood lead was due to petrol lead emissions.
4   If the current EPA petrol lead standards were removed, in 1983 there would be an estimated 134,000 black children with blood lead levels above 35 ug/dl which is normally considered to be a seriously high blood lead level.

The report stated:

We conclude from the results of the regression models and the statistical tests that there can be little doubt that petrol lead emissions are an important determinant, perhaps the most important single contributor, of the level of lead in blood.

The third study I have referred to was an isotopic lead experiment in north-west Italy where, in order to identify the input of petrol lead into blood, a lead of a different isotopic ratio was imported from the Broken Hill mine in Australia and added to petrol sold in the region. Initial results showed that 95% of lead in the area was the special lead, and about a quarter of the lead in blood of adults surveyed and 30% of lead in children was the special lead. This lead in blood has to be added to lead that has accumulated in the body, and also to lead from petrol from outside the sample area, to create a total picture of the body's lead burden and on the basis of the study it would appear that a 30% petrol lead input into our bodies represents the very minimum. Known as 'the Turin Study', it was partly sponsored by the EEC.

The British Debate
    As with the health question, the Ministerial and civil service 'bible' on sources of lead exposure has been the report of the Lawther Committee, and on this subject it has proved to be equally insupportable. While it acknowledged that 'about 90% of airborne lead is

derived from petrol', it concluded that the contribution from air lead to most people 'would be of the order of 10% and possibly a little more if allowance is made for intake of airborne lead via dust'. Inexplicably this Committee concluded that 'most people in the UK derive the major part of their lead body burden from food' but completely failed to identify where lead in food comes from. Food is not a *source* of lead exposure – it is a *route* whereby lead from a genuine source enters the body. Lead is not naturally in food. Not only did Lawther fail to say this but he actually said the opposite:

> We have seen that in the vast majority of the population airborne lead, including that derived from petrol, is usually a minor contributor to the body burden. Normally, food is the major source and we have seen no evidence that this is substantially enhanced by contamination by airborne lead.

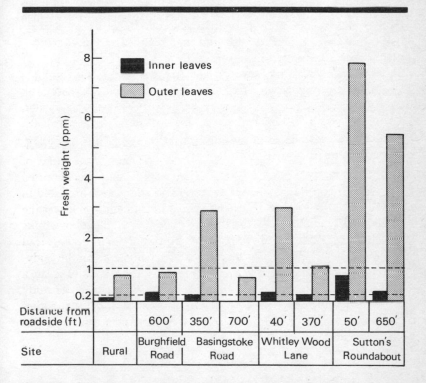

Figure 8   LEAD LEVELS in cabbage, Reading area. Data provided by Reading Environmental Health Department. The dotted lines at 1.0 and 0.2 ppm indicate the present UK statutory maxima for lead in most general food and infant food respectively. It can be seen that lead is greater in the outer leaves and thus the greater contamination is from the air, not the soil.

This aspect of the Lawther Report was also widely criticised at the time it was published. *Municipal Engineering and Environmental Technology* described it as 'bizarre'. Commenting on Lawther's claim that food represented 45–90% of the body burden of lead the magazine said, 'So far, so good. But the crucial unanswered question is where the lead in food comes from.' Sir Henry Yellowlees, in his famous letter, stated a year later that 'further evidence' had 'strongly' supported the view that 'lead in petrol is a major contributor to blood lead acting through the food chain as well as by inhalation'. There had in fact been little 'further' evidence; the evidence had already been there in vast quantities.

Figure 8 makes the point simply; it shows how the lead on the outer leaves of cabbages in Berkshire was far more substantial than the lead on the inner leaves; this supports the contention that the lead comes from air on to these plants rather than upwards from the soil.

Research has demonstrated that plant life in urban areas is much more contaminated with lead than plant life in rural areas; if plants received their lead naturally from the soil, this would not necessarily be so. It is, however, consistent with the fact that their lead intake comes largely from man-created sources; and notably from the air.

The whole issue of the sources of lead exposure was also explored at the CLEAR symposium in 1982, and by Professor Rutter in his summing-up.

He concluded:

> Taken as a whole the evidence clearly indicates that petrol accounts for a substantial proportion of the overall variance in environmental lead. Moreover, it may well be that petrol contributes more to the body burden of lead in early childhood than it does in adult life . . . although difficulties prevent any accurate estimate of the contribution of petrol to body lead, they fall far short of any serious distraction from the general thesis that it is a major, probably the major, contributor. Certainly it is apparent that the removal of lead from petrol would result in a significant and worthwhile reduction in environmental lead. It is important, too, to appreciate that much of the intake of lead from petrol does not occur through inhalation but through the ingestion of lead polluted food and dust. The implication is that living in a rural area away from motorways may not help as much as one thought.

He concluded that the Lawther Committee had 'very substantially underestimated the risks from lead in petrol'.

And so, having left the Lawther Committee far behind on the health hazard caused by low levels of exposure, Rutter had now abandoned it completely on the contribution of petrol lead.

It was more than fair that Rutter should emphasise not only lead in food but lead in dust; one man who has undertaken considerable research in this area is Mick Duggan of the Environmental Sciences Division of the Greater London Council. He supports with his studies the Rutter view that the route of dust-hand-mouth is a significant one for children and in a characteristically mild interpretation of highly-convincing data says:

> There is a *prima facie* case for the hypothesis that the ingestion of urban dust via dirty hands gives rise to a significant intake of lead during early childhood. The peak level of blood lead frequently observed at two to three years of age, the enhancement of the child-adult blood lead ratio which occurs in contaminated areas, and the relationship between blood lead in dust seen in many studies can all be accounted for by the hypothesis.

Duggan was one of those responsible for a GLC survey of 21 Inner London school playgrounds. Some of the levels were so high that the results were kept confidential to avoid frightening parents. Rick Rogers, education writer for the *New Statesman*, obtained the report and published it in April 1981. The readings varied from 120 ppm to a staggering 26,500 ppm. Rogers quoted the report as stating that 'There is . . . no doubt that petrol-derived lead is in general the main contributor to lead in urban dust'.

> The research also indicated that dust levels on the pavement were generally higher than the dust levels in playgrounds, suggesting that the lead was coming from the direction of the road, and thus the traffic, rather than from old paint on the school buildings.

In the 1978 report to the National Research Council in Canada on the effects of lead in that country, J. F. Jaworski stated:

> A number of studies implicate automotive lead as one of the major contributing factors to elevated lead levels in adults, and especially in children. In the case of children automotive lead is not only inhaled but is also ingested as settled dust in the home and in the playground.

It is noticeable that whilst the Lawther Committee was failing to note all these points, Jaworski was having no difficulty in doing so in Canada. For instance, on the question of the food chain:

> Fallout of airborne lead onto crops, especially near smelters and highways (the latter from leaded petrol) can contribute more to the total lead associated with the plant than can the soil. Horses and cattle

grazing near busy highways and lead smelters have consumed enough contaminated forage to induce overt signs of lead poisoning. . . . Although the fallout of airborne lead on plants may be washed off, leafy vegetables and rough-surfaced vegetables may retain most of this lead. Commercial frozen vegetables may be less well washed than those prepared fresh at home. There is some indication that lead and other heavy metals inhibit the uptake by plants of such nutrients as iron and potassium which are essential for proper animal and human nutrition.

The Royal Commission on Environmental Pollution received evidence from the major British research organisation with responsibility for studies on the physical and biological sciences relating to the natural environment, The Natural Environment Research Council (NERC). This important body reminded the Commission that 'the unofficial NERC policy for some years has been to argue in favour of reducing emissions of lead, especially from motor vehicles, on the principle that it is wrong to knowingly add to the burden of lead in man and the environment'.

It reported that the NERC has . . .

> invested considerable effort over the last decade in the study of the nature and origins of lead and other elements and reported that the weight of evidence indicates a widespread influence of anthropogenic lead upon concentrations of lead in the troposphere over much of the world, and a highly significant input of lead into the oceans.

After reviewing this work at considerable length it made a number of comments:

> It is sufficient to note . . . that motor vehicle emissions are major sources of lead contamination of soils and vegetation close to roadways. Some of this lead finds its way into the diet and, therefore, the bodies of man and other animals.
>
> Whilst further research is needed to determine accurately the nature and more subtle effects of lead in the environment, the weight of evidence indicates that lead from industrial sources and motor vehicles may cause contamination of the environment on a large scale. A substantial proportion of the lead in recent sediments of rivers, lakes, estuaries, and the seas, may be derived ultimately from petrol.

Despite this overwhelming evidence of a major input of lead in petrol to human beings, the Department of the Environment was still in 1982 stating that its 'view on sources and pathways of human uptake of environmental lead in the UK is at present principally based on the authoritative report of the DHSS working party . . . chaired by Professor Patrick Lawther'. The DOE, therefore, were clinging to the Lawther report with a tenacity only equalled by the

Associated Octel Company and in the face of overwhelming evidence that it was seriously flawed.

The DOE were still claiming that 'an adult in the normal range (8–15 ug/dl) living in an urban area, might be expected to derive about one fifth of his/her total exposure from petrol lead'. This position is indefensible in the context of the evidence I have outlined in this chapter.

What, in fact, is the contribution by petrol-lead to the lead in our bodies? The simple answer, as Professor Rutter has said, is that we do not exactly know, both because it varies according to our age, where we live, and a variety of other circumstances. But I suggest that any reasonable person studying the evidence will see that the 10% suggested by Lawther and the 10–20% enthusiastically parrotted by Whitehall and British Ministers in defence of their policies is an absurdity.

Were lead in petrol contributing 20% to lead in human beings, that would in any event be justification for action. Once we reach 30%, the figure suggested by the British Medical Association and supported by the Turin study, we unquestionably have cause for

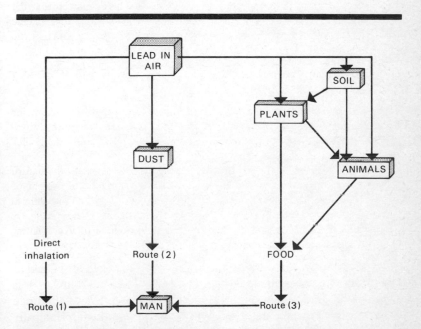

Figure 9 MAIN PATHWAYS of airborne lead to Man. Source: Robin Russell Jones, *Lead Versus Health*, 1983.

action. When we reach the 46% suggested by the US Environmental Protection Agency, the case for action has become extremely urgent. However, in their chapter in 'Lead Versus Health' Russell Jones and Stephens make a powerful case for an input of over 50% (and even the EPA acknowledges that for some city children in America the figure is over 60%). At this level the position of the British authorities on the issue is seen to be the height of irresponsibility.

It should be remembered that huge quantities of lead are blasted into the atmosphere from car exhausts all over the world year after year. This lead does not disappear into infinity. It descends somewhere, and accumulates year after year over wider and wider areas. One does not need to be a scientist to see that this must be so, and to conclude that we are slowly and steadily making the earth more and more dangerous to inhabit. Even if we are careless of our own fate, or that of our children, any thoughts at all for the generations to come should force the conclusion that continuing the practice of adding lead to petrol is creating an appalling legacy of pollution for them.

4.
How safe is safe?

THERE HAS been in Britain considerable monitoring of lead levels in air, dust, paint and water, as well as monitoring of blood lead levels. This research is, however, useless unless it can be sensibly evaluated, and this is only possible if the results are compared with realistic safety levels. Unfortunately, the authorities and the public have different priorities when it comes to safety levels

– the individual wants the bias to be towards his or her safety, while the authorities want the bias to be towards what they perceive as cost-effective or practical. Most of the so-called safety levels or thresholds for lead pollution have been determined for administrative and political convenience rather than on the basis of the medical or scientific evidence.

On June 30, 1982, the British Minister responsible for co-ordinating policies on lead pollution, Giles Shaw, illustrated how valuable an unrealistic safety threshold can be to his kind of politician. He reported on the 1981 UK survey implementing the EEC Directive on biological screening of the population for lead and demonstrated that of the 35 groups surveyed, mainly chosen for their higher-than-normal risk of exposure to lead pollution, 32 met the 'reference level' set in the Directive.

> Taken as a whole, the results reinforce the Government's view that levels of lead pollution in the environment give no cause for alarm.

The EEC 'reference levels' are as follows: 'if more than 50% of any groups surveyed exceeded 20 ug/dl, more than 10% exceeded 30 ug/dl, or more than 2% exceeded 35 ug/dl, the group is held to have breached the reference level in question'.

Shaw revealed that few people in the 35 groups monitored had blood lead levels above 35 ug/dl and this was the basis for his reassurance. However, even while he was making these claims, his own officials were preparing a circular to local authorities proposing a reduction in the action or safety level from 35 ug/dl to 25 ug/dl. As *The Guardian* reported a week later, 'a different picture emerges at the proposed 25 level. Preliminary results show that people in 31 of the 35 groups had lead levels about 20 ug/dl'.

In other words, by operating on an unrealistic safety threshold, Shaw had been able to claim that there was no serious problem, whereas at an equally unrealistic safety threshold of 25, *The Guardian* was able to show there was a considerable problem. I say 'equally unrealistic threshold' because the evidence of the last two chapters would suggest that this figure of 25 is at least double the real safety level, and this would have completely reversed all of the findings from the screening programme.

We have a situation where the EEC clearly sees 35 ug/dl as the danger point, the United States fixes it at 30, although there the maximum permissible population mean level is 15 ug/dl, and the United Kingdom at 25. Where does the truth lie? We know the British Medical Association's view from its evidence to the Royal Commission:

For operational and regulatory purposes it would be desirable to set levels or zones of lead considered dangerous, unacceptable, acceptable, or safe, but there is little justification for such a classification on biological or toxicological grounds.

The BMA thus supports the CLEAR position, namely that there are no medical and scientific grounds for the official safety threshold. Until such time as the authorities abandon unrealistic safety levels, all monitoring of blood lead levels will not only be fruitless but counter-productive, for politicians like Shaw, by employing exaggerated safety levels, can actually use them to avoid introducing appropriate protective measures.

What, then, is a realistic safety threshold? The answer is that we still don't know enough to fix one precisely. We do, however, know enough *not* to fix one. The implication is that we have to take defensive action at the lowest levels where ill-effects have been convincingly demonstrated and the evidence suggests that such a level would have to be under 10 ug/dl.

It is easy to see why the politicians resist this suggestion for it could mean that Sir Henry Yellowlees' figure of 'hundreds of thousands' of children at risk is still an under-estimate – it could literally be millions. Furthermore, a maximum figure of 10 ug/dl would mean that the authorities in Britain have maintained a safety threshold of 3½ times the realistically maximum figure until just recently, and even now operate on the basis of 2½ times the realistic maximum. No wonder they have been able to get away with inadequate lead protection policies.

In Britain there are no statutory limits for lead in air, lead in water, lead in dust, or lead in paint, yet these are the main routes for lead entry to the body. There are guidelines and recommendations but, of course, without statutory controls, no-one has recourse in law if standards are ignored.

Lead in Air
Britain has accepted the EEC standard for lead in air of 2 ug/m³ or 8 ug/m³ near heavy traffic, despite the fact that the United States' figure is 1.5 ug/m³ and the GLC guideline is 1 ug/m³. Once more we have a considerable discrepancy between standard-setters. The natural level of lead in the air is 0.0004 ug/m³.

Lead in Dust
The GLC action level is 5,000 ppm (parts per million), the DOE

guideline 2,000 ppm, the GLC's 'ideal safety level' 500 ppm, but the natural level of lead in dust is 15 ppm.

No wonder there was uproar in London in 1979 when 28 Inner London primary schools were tested for lead pollution and, the *New Statesman*, reported at the time, produced some staggering results:

Four primary schools are so polluted by lead and other metals that they are causing the Inner London Education Authority 'extreme concern'. . . . Telferscot in Balham, SW12 (5190 ppm*); Rushmore in Clapton E5 (4730); and Harbinger in Cahir Street E14 (3150) recorded a dangerously high mean level of concentration of lead in dust. The readings at these schools ranged from 120 ppm up to a staggering 26,500 ppm.
The other lead-risk schools in the survey are:
Henry Compton, Kingswood Road, SW6 (1990 ppm); Pakeman, Hornsey Road N7 (1840); Bentworth, Bentworth Road W12 (1800); St. Thomas More, Appleton Road SE9 (1350); Redriff, Rotherhithe Street SE16 (1100); Penton, Richie Street N1 (1010); Dulwich Village Infants, Dulwich SE21 (940); Seven Mills, Malabar Street, E14 (890); St. Stephen's, Westbourne Park Road W2 (890); Latchmere, Burns Road SW11 (880); Drayton Park, N5 (880); Phoenix, Bow Road E3 (880); Boxgrove, Boxgrove Road, SE2 (860); Paddington Green, Park Place Village W2 (740); St. Saviours, Lewisham High Street, SE13 (710); Parliament Hill, Highgate Road, NW5 (700); Our Lady's Convent, Amhurst Park, N16 (660); Brockley, Beecroft Road, SE4 (520); George Elliot, Marlborough Hill, NW8 (510); Beechcroft, Beechcroft Road, SW17 (500).

In late 1982, sampling of lead in dust in school playgrounds in Hammersmith and Fulham produced further disturbing results. Of 12 schools surveyed only one had dust lead levels below the GLC guideline of 500 ppm. Others had figures ranging from 535 to a staggering 10,300. This last school had a range of findings from 1,550 to a terrifying 85,550.

Lead in Food

This is the one area where there is a statutory safety level. This is 0.2 ppm for tinned food for babies, and 1 ppm for tinned food for adults. The natural level of lead in food would be 0.002 ppm.

Lead in Paint

All paint sold in the United States is limited to 600 ppm of lead by law. In Britain, paint used on toys is limited to 2,500 ppm, the

*ppm = parts per million

EEC maximum for lead in paint is 5,000 ppm, and the UK maximum for lead in paint is 10,000 ppm. (This is done in Britain by voluntary agreement with the paint manufacturers who, as in the case of the lead additive manufacturers, disclaim any health risk from their product.) Paints with greater levels than this are supposed to carry a public health warning to the effect that the contents should not be used on surfaces liable to be chewed or sucked by children.

Lead in Water

The WHO guideline is 100 ug/1 (micrograms) and the EEC guideline is 50 ug/l. It has been calculated that for the mean blood lead level of the population not to exceed 15 ug/dl, the water supply should contain no more than 10 ug/l of lead. The natural level of lead in water would be 0.02 ug/l.

It will be clear from the above that there is no uniformity between countries on safety levels and thresholds, and complete inconsistency in Britain. Furthermore, the lack of statutory imposition of safety levels indicates the lack of will to eliminate lead pollution. A DOE circular to local authorities in 1982 was widely criticised for the weakness of its advice and instructions.

This brief look at some of the safety levels or thresholds also explains why the authorities are anxious to maintain them at the highest possible point; as more local authorities and educational authorities begin to carry out monitoring activities, and produce the kind of figures for lead in dust and paint found in London schools, so public concern rises, and with it the need for more public expenditure to eliminate old paint, replace old water pipes, and ban lead in petrol.

We urgently need a re-evaluation of all safety levels and standards with an emphasis on prudence rather than administrative convenience. At present the answer to the question 'How safe is safe?' is that all the levels the authorities claim to be safe are undoubtedly unsafe, and the perpetuation of policies based on these levels is therefore the height of irresponsibility.

5.
Down to 0.15

Lead in petrol first became a political issue in Britain in 1971 when Professor Derek Bryce-Smith of Reading University published a paper in *Chemistry in Britain* describing lead pollution as 'a growing hazard to public health' and pinpointing lead in petrol as a significant source of exposure. Unquestionably he did more than anyone else to arouse public concern about lead in petrol. In the earlier years, when his claims of a health hazard were rejected more arbitrarily than they are now, he was often isolated, and perhaps yielded to the temptation to raise his voice to be heard, only to be trapped in a vicious circle whereby the less that people listened, the louder he would shout, thus alienating them still further. Sometimes, too, he would appear to extend his case beyond a point that the evidence would justify. Perhaps his most controversial step was to offer evidence to the Scarman enquiry into the Brixton riots in London laying at least part of the blame for the riots on the effects of lead pollution. For all we know, one day he may be proved correct; however, the scientific grounds for the claim did not justify the risk he took of public scorn.

It would have been less than objective not to mention these points, but they do not detract from his courage and persistence and from the fact that his basic claim – that lead in petrol was a health hazard – was fully justified.

Another who became concerned about lead pollution in the late Sixties was the science writer, Anthony Tucker. He wrote a major *Guardian* article in 1967 and later included a chapter in his 1972 book *The Toxic Metals*. In it he argued that of all the known dangerous environmental contaminants in developed countries, the levels of lead – as measured in the blood of ordinary people – were the highest. He challenged the safety thresholds as 'bogus', and questioned whether researchers were 'cooking the books'. This is a typical passage:

> By taking virtually every assumption that would minimise the calculated intake of lead from the atmosphere, for instance, and the word 'assumption' needs to be stressed, Britain's Medical Research Council Air Pollution Unit arrived at the reassuring conclusion that even for individuals working in the busiest streets for eight hours a day the elimination of lead from petrol would reduce their daily lead absorption by only 7%. Within weeks of the first announcement of this result in January 1971, it had been quoted five times by Ministers and frequently by petroleum spokesmen.

The Head of the Medical Research Council's Air Pollution Unit at this time was Professor Patrick Lawther.

As a result of the Bryce-Smith and Tucker disclosures, the issue was taken up by a Conservative Peer, Lord O'Hagan. Tucker in his book illustrates the failure of politicians to take the issue seriously at that time by recalling a particularly ludicrous discussion in the House of Lords in March 1971:

> LORD O'HAGAN: My Lords, I beg leave to ask the Question which stands in my name on the order paper (To ask her Majesty's Government what they intend to do about lead in petrol).

> LORD MOWBRAY & STOUGHTON: I told the noble Lord on March 10, H.M. Government are considering whether any action is needed to reduce the lead content of petrol.

> LORD O'HAGAN: . . . Does he accept that catalysts in after-burners are poisoned by lead? And even if he is not able to accept that, will he publish the evidence on which he based his earlier and rather complacent reply?

> LORD M & S: . . . Catalysts used in America for the after-burners are poisoned by lead. May I ask the noble Lord to repeat his second question?

> LORD O'HAGAN: . . . Will the noble Lord publish the evidence on which he based his views?

LORD M & S: . . . The evidence on which I based my information was worked out by the Medical Research Council, as I informed him. I can absolutely vouch for its accuracy.

LORD O'HAGAN: . . . Is the noble Lord saying that what is poisonous in America is not poisonous here?

LORD M & S: No, my Lords. What I said is that the catalyst is destroyed by the presence of lead in petrol. . . .

LORD SHACKLETON: My Lords, is the noble Lord aware that I think the House is nearly as confused as he is by his answer? I wonder whether he would now take advice from the noble Lord, Lord O'Hagan, and choose an opportunity to speak again . . . ?

LORD AMULREE: My Lords, surely the issue is whether the amount of lead in petrol which comes out of exhaust fumes . . . is likely to be deleterious to health.

LORD M & S: . . . We accept that lead in itself is not a good thing to have: we are not going to give ourselves more. What we must also realise, though, is that even the natives in New Guinea have an enormous intake of lead. The amount of extra lead we get from pollution by exhaust gases is comparatively small. I accept that we would be better without it, but if we do without it we have to use a lower octane petrol . . . it is a matter of economics and sense.

LORD HENLEY: My Lords, how will this affect the lead in the noble Lord's pencil?

LORD SHACKLETON: . . . Is the noble Lord aware that he has made a very serious statement. I understand that there are cannibals in New Guinea. Is he aware that there is already concern about the edibility of Western people because of the amount of DDT in them? How do DDT and lead mix? Is this not a matter for the Food and Agriculture Office?

LORD M & S: My Lords, I can assure the noble Lord the leader of the Opposition that we are not importing any cannibal meat from New Guinea.

Three other 1971 events are worth recording:

First, a number of newspapers reported the leak of a confidential document circulated within the Mobil Oil Corporation by its Corporate Management Sciences Program in the United States and sent to the Chairman of Mobil in Britain. Its summary stated:

Lead should be removed from petrol because it contributes to engine deposits, causes particulate exhaust emissions, increases hydrocarbon emission, is a dangerous heavy metal poison and destroys the effectiveness of catalytic converters. These reasons for removal justify an immediate effort to reduce the average lead content of petrol.

The cover of the report said the contents:

must not be disclosed or discussed with any person outside.

The Sunday Times commented:

In total opposition to the bland public announcements of some oil companies on the subject, it confirms all that environmentalists have been saying recently about the dangers of lead in petrol.

Then there were a series of comments by Peter Walker, then in charge of the DOE, which suggested growing concern in Whitehall.

On April 21 he stated: 'I am advised that the levels of lead in the environment do not endanger health.'

On July 20 he stated: 'I have recently commissioned further measurements of lead in the urban atmosphere.'

On August 3, he reported nine studies into the problem of lead pollution.

On October 20, he said that although the Chief Medical Officer had not found evidence that atmospheric lead was hazardous to health, nevertheless, he thought it advisable to halt the rising trend and possibly reverse it. He also admitted that this trend largely resulted from the increase in motor vehicles and that possible action was being considered.

On November 21 he stated that he hoped to announce further controls over pollution from motor vehicles he thought necessary, and that he was paying particularly close attention to the use of lead additives in fuel.

Finally, in December, Yellowlees' predecessor, Dr. G. E. Godber, Chief Medical Officer at the DHSS, wrote to all medical officers of health on the question of environmental hazards from lead. Despite the Walker comments, this was an extraordinarily complacent letter. There was, Godber said, no evidence that the intake of lead at average levels in Britain had any adverse effects. Lead in the atmosphere was in extremely small concentrations and there was no 'general hazard from this source at the present levels of emission'. He was equally complacent on other areas of exposure and ended 'there is nothing in this information to suggest more than a planned review of conditions in any affected part of your own area but you will no doubt wish to put this in hand now'.

In January 1972 the British public were made more aware of the toxic qualities of lead by news that the Imperial Smelting

Corporation's lead and zinc plant at Avonmouth would have to be closed for several months because it had been poisoning its workers and endangering nearby residents. More than 100 employees were found to have exceptionally high levels of lead in their blood.

Soil and plants in the area were contaminated and horses had died after eating lead-poisoned grass. A TUC medical adviser was quoted in *The Sunday Times* as saying the plant 'leaked lead at every pore'. The local council rejected planning permission for a housing estate a mile from the smelter because of health risks. Of lead levels, the *Sunday Times* article ended with a prophetic remark: 'Tragically, history may yet show that there is no safe level.'

In 1972 those who were to remain on different sides of the debate ten years later were already to be seen in public confrontation at a conference organised by the Institute of Petroleum in London. Lawther and Dr. Donald Barltrop both presented papers calculated to quieten fears, and Dr. Patrick Barry of Associated Octel supported them in discussion. Bryce-Smith and Stephens lined up on the other side, challenging both the Lawther and Barltrop papers.

Close scrutiny of the record of the debate shows that Lawther's MRC Air Pollution Unit consistently followed the same line and was equally consistently criticised. For instance, after it offered evidence to the public inquiry on the proposed West Cross motorway, stating that there was little difference in blood-lead levels between taxi drivers on a three-hour day shift and those on a three-and-a-half hour night shift and drawing the conclusion that airborne lead from traffic did not significantly affect human blood-lead levels, a doctor from Middlesex Hospital Medical School wrote to *The Lancet* to point out that the short term day and night differences would be swamped by the exposure all the drivers would be subjected to during normal urban living throughout any 24 hours. The MRC conclusions were invalid or called for qualification.

Even then Lawther and his colleagues at the MRC were defining food as the main source of lead in man without defining where the lead came from. The Middlesex doctor, Dr. R. M. Hicks, wrote: 'Since no information is given about lead exposure either in food or atmosphere of the two groups of drivers in their non-taxi-driving hours, the observations are not relevant.' She expressed concern that 'these untenable conclusions will be cited by those in favour of retaining lead in petrol'.

On June 6, 1973, *The Sunday Mercury* in Birmingham quoted that city's environmental health officer as suggesting that warning labels should be published on all petrol pumps. He was quoted as saying:

I take the view that when a toxic substance is sold to the public it ought to be declared. If people are increasingly aware of the dangers of lead, they may eventually turn to buying new brands of petrol which would be lead-free. It is possible to produce perfectly satisfactory petrol without this lead additive.

In 1974 the oil companies voluntarily accepted a restriction to 0.55 grams per litre and, although this was a nonsense because they were already using considerably less lead in petrol than this, it contributed to the issue fading from the public gaze until 1976 when in an article in *The Sunday Times* on January 11, 1976, Mark Ottaway and Anthony Terry reported:

On January 1 the legal limit of lead in petrol in Germany was reduced to 0.15 grams per litre, well below the limit anywhere else in Western Europe and the 0.40 grams per litre below which the DOE accept British industry cannot reasonably be asked to go. The current legal limit in this country is 0.64 grams per litre though, in November 1974, the Government obtained a voluntary agreement from the oil companies to restrict themselves to 0.55 grams per litre. This was a sham. No petrol, not even 5-star, had more than that in 1974, when the average lead content of all petrol sold was 0.52 grams per litre. In 1971 it was 0.46 grams per litre. In banning lead for health reasons, the Bonn Government rode roughshod over the objections of the oil companies and of its fellow EEC members. These were identical to the ones which swayed the DOE. All have turned out to be either false or exaggerated.

Oil companies throughout the world have been unanimous on the perils of what Germany has done. These are:

(1) *Increased petrol consumption. False:* tests carried out by the West German Motoring Association show that fuel consumption on the new low-lead petrol is the same as before.

(2) *Extensive modification of existing cars. False:* in West Germany, when £90 'leadless petrol adaptation kits' were offered to motorists, the Motoring Association found that a few models needed a slight advance in their ignition timing. That was all. Leyland cars are making no changes in the models they sell there. Our Moscow reporter has never had any problem running his standard Wolseley on lead-free petrol in the Soviet Union.

(3) *A considerable increase in the price of petrol. False:* there has been no increase in the price of German petrol, despite initial scare stories of a 25p per gallon increase. The German companies say they may eventually have to increase prices by between a penny and twopence a gallon to recoup their costs in new refining equipment, and the fact that more crude oil is needed to produce a given amount of low-lead petrol.

(4) *Massive outlay on new refineries and increased oil imports. False:* the effects of these appear to have been exaggerated. . . . West German oil imports are expected to go up by not more than 5% compared with the DOE estimate of 10% for totally lead-free petrol. Again, not a major discrepancy. *But* (their emphasis) the extra oil is not lost; most is recovered in valuable by-products and the investment programme must be considered in the light of normal capital expenditure.
Perhaps this explains why German petrol has not increased in price.

(5) *Excessive wear and tear on engines. Unlikely:* German petrol companies are now fervent in their assurances to motorists that the new petrol will not harm their engines as they once were in their threat that it would.

The whole article was appropriately headed 'The Great Lead Petrol Lie'.

In 1978 the issue re-emerged in the forefront of public attention and has stayed there ever since. First, Dr. A. C. Chamberlain, working at the Atomic Energy Research Authority's laboratories in Harwell, produced a report that was not published for two months until it was sent to a University in America and from there forwarded to a British journalist who passed it on to Jeff Rooker, MP. With the support of five other scientists, Chamberlain reported that the intake into the human body from airborne lead was three times the level they had estimated in an earlier 1975 report.

Also in 1978, three parents with children living in the centre of London took British Petroleum, Shell, Associated Octel, and the Ford Motor Company to court to claim damages for 'nuisance, assault, and negligence in that these petrol processors and car manufacturers are causing brain damage to our children by poisoning the atmosphere with lead additives'. The driving force behind this action was Nicholas Albery, then an architect's assistant, sueing on behalf of his son. The lower court found there was 'reasonable cause of action' and on April 15, 1980, the case came before the Court of Appeal. The children, or their representatives, were able to produce evidence of high lead levels in air and dust in the area, and also in vegetables grown in their gardens. They were also able to demonstrate elevated lead levels in their children. The plaintiffs asked for arbitration and £60 damages, later reduced to £1 plus £1 special damages in an attempt to avoid costs. The defendants applied for the proceedings to be struck out as 'frivolous and vexatious' and showing no reasonable cause of action.

Nicholas Albery testified that he believed his child to be 'damaged by the defendants'. He said:

To other parents, and nursery attendants and people who know Merlyn well, these signs of damage are evident and were evident before lead was known to be the cause. The signs of this damage are hyperactivity, fit-like tantrums, undue unruliness. Tests on his hair lead level have confirmed this damage, in that his lead level is very high indeed, many times over the lead level of those children whom researchers have found to be in the adversely-affected range.

Eleanora Budden, the mother of another child in the case, testified that her son had been exceptionally irritable as a baby, had no ability to concentrate, and the investigations revealed that he had high lead levels.

I think it should be made clear that the case is not about money, but about preventing further damage to children, including my own child. I feel that no sum of money can truly compensate him for the damage he has suffered.

The case ended when Lord Justice Magaw read a judgement that the action had no real chance of success and that it was the duty of the court to put an end to this action. He stated:

Manufacturers or suppliers of petrol could not be negligent in a matter such as this where there cannot be varied limits for varied circumstances, if the limit to which they adhered was the limit which they were entitled reasonably to be consistent within the public interest.

Weight was given to the fact that Parliament had laid down limits and that the defendants had complied with them.

The authority of Parliament must prevail. Where Parliament has decided a matter of general policy, the courts cannot properly be asked to make decisions, by way of litigation under the adversary procedure, the effect of which would, or might, be that the courts would lay down, and require to be enforced with the authority of the courts, a different and inconsistent policy. We stress that this does not mean that where Parliament prescribes a limit the courts may not hold a defendant liable for negligence even though he does not go above that limit. But that does not arise where what the court is asked to do, as here, is to lay down a limit which must necessarily be of general application, inconsistent with the limit of general application prescribed under the authority of Parliament, by reference to the selfsame criterion as Parliament has applied.

Thus the industries were now able to continue the process of polluting safe in the knowledge that if they could persuade Whitehall and then Westminster to accept safety levels satisfactory to them, there was no possibility of prosecution or of civil damages. Whether or not this is sound law, let alone justice, what is reprehensible about the attitude of industry is that provided they are covered by laws or regulations they seem to feel no *moral* obligation or responsibility. A criminal who on a technicality is found innocent may well celebrate with gusto in his local pub that night, but even he does not live a life of such self-delusion as to believe the technicality protecting his freedom makes him any less criminal!

It is, incidentally, ironic that one of the initial aims of the court action was to seek an injunction to force the companies to reduce lead levels in petrol to 0.15 grams per litre; this level has subsequently become law.

(There was an extraordinary sequel to this case two years later, when Shell and BP were allowed £33,000 from the Legal Aid Fund towards their costs. Initially they claimed £50,000 but the Law Society objected and it was subsequently reduced. The intention of the Legal Aid Fund is to enable those in genuine need to defend themselves. The Law Society were quoted as saying in *The Guardian*, 'We have done our best to safeguard the Fund, but the Court of Appeal overruled us'.)

At 5.37 am at the end of an all-night sitting on August 1, 1978, Jeff Rooker, Member of Parliament for Birmingham, Perry Barr, raised the issue in the House of Commons. 'In the whole of the debate which has gone on for years we have had deafening silence from the oil companies' he said. He continued:

> They did not enter the debate. The most that they are prepared to say these days is that they will do, or comply with, whatever the Government requires them to do. That is not a very satisfactory attitude for the companies to adopt, because we are here dealing with some of the most powerful organisations in the world, more powerful than many national Governments. . . . They are able to move power and capital around the world, and are sometimes involved in toppling Governments. . . . One sometimes questions whether the Department of the Environment at Marsham Street is really up to dealing with these organisations. I submit that it is not.

He suggested that there was

> plenty of evidence from people with no financial axe to grind that we may have to wait for a catastrophe, like an open dropping of IQ levels, before action is taken.

In reply Kenneth Marks, Under-Secretary at the DOE, said the studies were contradictory. It was still generally accepted that the normal upper limit for lead in blood is 'taken to be 35 ug/dl'. The average level in the population was about 20 ug/dl, well beneath the accepted upper limit. The research that had so far been done on sources of lead in man 'indicate that most people's lead intake comes mainly from food and drink.' (Yet another politician thus failed to question how the lead entered 'food and drink'.)

He emphasised that Ministers were committed to a programme of reduction of lead to 0.4 grams per litre from January 1, 1981 in line with the then EEC directive.

> We recognise that further action will be required and we are already considering what the next step should be to maintain or reduce the level below the 1971 level.
>
> We have been accused of ignoring the evidence said to link lead in petrol with serious health risk. We reject the criticism of complacency. It is right that there should be concern about lead pollution. It is right that people wish to be assured that there is not significant danger to them and their children. . . . It is the Government's business to ensure that their reasonable and legitimate concerns are met by appropriate action. However, it is also the Government's business to ensure that expensive measures are justified by evidence or reasonable hypotheses about the source, levels and effects of lead.
>
> It would not be reasonable to embark on a very expensive series of measures unless we had good reason to believe that those measures were necessary. A balance needs to be struck.

Also in August 1978 four scientists at Great Ormond Street Hospital who have (perhaps with the exception of one) always maintained an ultra-critical line on the evidence of the relationship between lead and neuropsychological dysfunction in children, Professor Barbara Clayton, Professor Philip Graham, H. T. Delves, Senior Lecturer, and Richard Lansdown, Chief Psychologist, wrote an extraordinary paper at the behest of the DHSS criticising the David and Needleman studies. Their critique was widely circulated in Whitehall, and used to suggest to Ministers that this US research was unreliable.

These four scientists had, however, broken with basic scientific practice in two-respects: first, they had not contacted either David or Needleman to obtain the full details of their studies. Second, they did not in the first instance submit their comments and criticisms to David and Needleman to offer them the opportunity of correcting any misinterpretations or misunderstandings – quite apart from the fact that it is established scientific courtesy to so do.

Unfortunately for both the DHSS and the four scientists, their document typed on Great Ormond Street paper was leaked.

Whilst they acknowledged at one point that the Needleman paper 'was presented at a meeting and therefore was perhaps not as full as the published version', they nevertheless felt free to condemn it on a number of grounds. They also criticised David heavily. One sentence, however, states 'no information on other variables related to the results is given'. To other scientists reading this paper it seemed extraordinary that the four Great Ormond Street scientists should not have sought such additional information before taking such a cavalier attitude towards this work. Their response raised a very serious question as to their ability to reach objective and informed opinions on the research. Needless to say, the American scientists took considerable exception to this behaviour.

As a result of criticisms in the House of Commons, the four scientists wrote to *The Lancet* to state 'We prepared a report which was critical but adequate appraisal was difficult because full details of the work had not been published'. (This was a concession they had not adequately made in the initial document.) 'We should have sent copies to the workers who had delivered the papers; they do now have copies.' Needleman replied:

> Clayton et al are right to refer to difficulties of appraisal; the only written report of my group's work at that time was a 250 word abstract. Yet they faulted our study primarily because it overlooked certain variables reflecting parental attainment and neglect. In fact, these important variables were the subject of particular and extensive scrutiny, and I would have been pleased to share these data (now published in the full paper) with Clayton et al had they asked me to. It seems to me that the task of criticising another's work implies an obligation to obtain maximum information before issuing an evaluation.
> The British and American postal systems are often the subject of abuse but they periodically work. In October, two months after the critique of Clayton et al was distributed, I received two copies by air mail from UK colleagues but none from Clayton et al.
> A subject as significant to the public health as low level lead and brain function deserves careful and open review. I hope that all students of the subject will judge the conclusions of my group's work, and that of others, on the basis of the fully published record.

The fact that the four scientists still did not see the point was demonstrated by a follow-up letter by Professor Graham:

> It has already been acknowledged that he should have been sent a copy of the comments prepared for the DHSS *once it had been agreed these could be circulated more widely*, and I should like to repeat my regret that this did not happen.

Graham, thus, still would not acknowledge that he and his colleagues simply did not have sufficient information about the study to make a critique that would be fed into the policy-making machine and circulated widely, nor did he seem to concede that he had a duty to allow the two American scientists to comment *before* the document was submitted to the DHSS at all.

Given that Clayton and Lansdown were subsequently to be on the Lawther Committee, this episode could not but add to concern about its objectivity.

In a letter to a British colleague, Needleman reported on a meeting he had had with Dr. Graham:

> I expressed some doubt about the collegiality of not sharing his critical writings on my work while they were being distributed at large. . . . I continue to be puzzled by why I was not contacted by the Great Ormond Street group in the first place, why I was not sent a copy of the comments by them in the second place, and finally why the comments are addressed to no-one in particular.

On March 7, 1979, Jeff Rooker asked the Secretary of State for Social Services 'if his department paid a fee for the report requested from the Hospital for Sick Children, Great Ormond Street, . . . and if he will make a statement.'

Roland Moyle: No

On December 12, 1978, the subject was before the House of Commons once more, this time raised by Mrs. Joyce Butler, Labour MP for Wood Green. She quoted the findings of Needleman and Winneke, and called for more urgent action than a drop to 0.40 grams per litre by January 1, 1982. Having discussed other forms of exposure to lead, she concluded that:

> As so many of these traditional sources of lead hazard to children will remain it is even more important to tackle the one task that poses no real technical problem, namely the complete removal of lead from petrol, rather than to argue, as successive Ministers have done, that because it is only one source of lead pollution we should not regard it as a matter of urgency . . . the Secretary of State for Transport has said that studies are being put in hand to estimate the cost of possible longer-term options for further reducing emissions from petrol. I hope that he will balance beside those costs the total economic cost of a national IQ deficit of several points attributable to lead and the cost of lead-related behaviour disorders to society. If this were done, the scales would indicate that the costs of using lead-free petrol, whatever they might be, would be cheap at the price.

In the same debate Jeff Rooker raised the question of the research undertaken by Chamberlain at the United Kingdom Atomic Energy Authority at Harwell on behalf of the petroleum industry and the International Lead Zinc Research Organisation. He questioned whether this work should be unpublished.

I do not believe that industrial sponsors ought to be able to do this. It is not as if they are dealing with new products; we are talking about public health and the public interest. Harwell are constantly employed by Associated Octel to undertake research. This is believed to be very expensive. When one questions this, Ministers, civil servants and other scientists fall over themselves to emphasise that there can be no question about the integrity of Harwell. The fact remains that Associated Octel, whose record of distortion of the evidence I will review shortly, seem extremely happy with the results they receive from Harwell.

Rooker then questioned the detail of the Harwell research report:

Given that they came up with a figure three times greater than they had come up with before, and given that there were at least three factors in the report which combined to make them grossly under-estimate the figure that they had come up with before, what are we left with? We are left with a figure that no-one can trust. It is three times greater than their previous figure, and based on this estimate, there is a good chance that it may be even higher. Cognizance has to be taken of that.

On the setting up of the Lawther Committee, he asked whether the Minister would publish full details of all members drawing attention to any who had been involved in research wholly or partly sponsored by private industry.

If these people are to make up the working party, and if what they say is to be the basis of Government policy, it is legitimate to ask whether any of them have been involved in work wholly or partly sponsored by private industry.

Rooker went on to say:

It has been put to me that the composition of the working party gives grounds for belief that this exercise is more political than medical or scientific. That is a serious accusation to make against a high-powered committee, but it is a challenge that has to be met with substantive answers.

He questioned why Professor A. Goldberg, the Regius Professor of Medicine at the University of Glasgow who was involved in studies of lead pollution of considerable importance, was omitted.

Rooker then went on to deal with the paper produced by the four scientists from Great Ormond Street Hospital.

I understand that Great Ormond Street was told that it could distribute the paper to those requesting it. Why was that? I understand that it is the oil companies that are requesting the paper and quoting it in defence of putting lead in petrol. How did companies know that the paper had been prepared unless they were told by the DHSS or one of the four authors? It is bad enough that the courtesy was not extended to inform the American authors of the comments made in the paper. . . . The background to the paper is far more significant than the Harwell report. It is of significance because it is being used by the oil companies, organisations that have a direct interest. The four authors . . . have been used in a propaganda exercise by a Government department and the oil companies. Clearly they have been used. Their work has upset international colleagues because of the discourtesy that has been shown. It has made others suspicious because of the way in which the paper was put out.

Denis Howell, the responsible Minister, challenged Rooker for questioning the behaviour of the consultants. Rooker replied:

Here we go again. The same old twaddle is trotted out. I am not attacking the integrity of the authors. I am claiming that to protect their integrity someone has to say that they have been used in a public relations exercise. The Government have mis-used them. . . . The Government are hiding behind a pre-eminent hospital.

Nigel Spearing, Labour MP for Newham, South (and remember these are *Labour* MP's questioning a *Labour* Minister, and thus there was no party political advantage to be obtained) supported Rooker. Of his speech, Spearing said:

I suspect that the reason why he went into so much fascinating detail was that he knew that unless he did it would not get on the record at all. In this matter, as in so many others, the Government has not been very open. Backbenchers and members of the public, speaking without detailed knowledge, have had to drag out the facts bit by bit and part by part over the past four or five years.

Spearing revealed that the DHSS then still believed it was possible to achieve 'conclusive' evidence. He read an extract from a letter signed by the Secretary of State containing the sentence 'Research undertaken in the past has been carefully reviewed by British and international groups of experts whose advice was that the results were not conclusive.'

Denis Howell, Minister of State at the DOE, then replied to the debate. He recorded research and work that had taken place over the years on achieving voluntary restraints on lead in paint and regulations on lead in toys and pottery glazes. He pointed out that two statutory reductions in lead content of petrol had been made since 1976 and a third would limit to 0.40 grams per litre on January 1, 1981.

The object of the programme is to ensure that in spite of increased car use the total emission of lead is contained at the 1971 level.

He said that in 1975 the total lead used in petrol in Britain was 10,600 tonnes and that in 1978 it should be reduced to 10,000 tonnes.

I say without complacency that it needs to be emphasised that the average amount of lead in the bloodstream for the general population is 20 ug against the 35 ug of the WHO.

Howell was thus building his defence on the same indefensible safety threshold of 35 ug/dl that was later to be adopted by Conservative Ministers.

He then came back once more to the concept of conclusive evidence.

The view of (our) medical advisers and other experts – including the four consultants and specialists of Great Ormond Street Hospital, who are people of the highest calibre and integrity – is that the studies are far from conclusive.

Howell also showed that, at this stage anyway, he had failed completely to consider how lead entered food and water. Of the Harwell report he said:

The report's further conclusion was 'for the majority of rural and urban residents, the contribution of air lead to total lead intake is less than 10%.' Although that bears out the Government's conclusion that we are absorbing 90% of our lead from food and water, this is still an area of considerable concern.

Howell then devoted the rest of his speech to the alleged cost of eliminating lead from petrol.

The costs should be of the following kinds, in differing degrees or permutations, depending on whether octane levels are maintained: first, the cost of extra crude oil needed to produce high octane petrol; secondly, the investment costs of refineries to cope with more severe refining; thirdly, the additional consumption of petrol if the quality is reduced; fourthly, the investment in manufacturing costs in production of modified engines.

In May of that year the DOE published the report of a joint working party on lead pollution around Birmingham's Spaghetti Junction. While it demonstrated elevated lead levels, it was complacent about their effects. One member of the working party, Dr. Robert Stephens, broke ranks and stated he believed it was too complacent.

Bob Stephens, a Reader in Chemistry at Birmingham University, has for at least 12 years been a dedicated if self-effacing contributor to anti-lead campaigns in Britain. He has devoted most of those years to a detailed study of the scientific literature on lead and his input of knowledge and scientific integrity has been invaluable to CLEAR. He now forged a partnership with the more mercurial Bryce-Smith and they in turn involved the Conservation Society. This set up a working party whose driving force was Jill Runnette, a Wimbedon housewife. This organisation, the Campaign Against Lead in Petrol (CALIP) was to lead the fight for a number of years. Its first symposium was held in 1978.

As a result of the developing concern, Labour Minister, Denis Howell, announced the setting up of the DHSS working party under the chairmanship of Lawther. Once more the issue faded temporarily from the public attention whilst the working party deliberated. Then in 1980 word began to emerge of Lawther's conclusions – of the renewed faith in a threshold of 35 ug/dl, the playing down of the importance of lead in petrol, the brushing aside of the work of Needleman and others, and the rest.

In the meantime CALIP organised a further symposium addressed by Needleman from the United States and Winneke from Germany on their latest studies. The Society sent invitations to every member of the Lawther Committee. Not one of them attended, nor, according to the two, did they make any attempt to meet with Needleman or Winneke while they were in London.

Now magazine in January leaked Lawther's conclusions and warned 'It is a verdict that flies in the face of a mass of apparently contrary evidence from around the world as well as in Britain'. It quoted Lord Avebury – formerly Eric Lubbuck, the Liberal MP – the President of the Conservation Society as saying the working party was 'unrepresentative of medical opinion' and Conservative MP, Archie Hamilton, as saying 'There are a number of experts who have strong views about the dangers of lead in petrol who are not on it. It is a very unbalanced working party'. Denis Howell, who when in power had set up the working party, was quoted as finding it 'astonishing and disturbing'. There was also an extraordinary quote from Lawther on the subject of the Billick study. Although the findings 'looked spectacular', Lawther had written, 'There had to be some explanation and indeed we found it. I can assure you that the correlations so dramatically portrayed can be explained without reference to petrol at all'. Billick was quoted as replying that Lawther's comments could not be justified as they stood. 'I can answer scientific statements but not religious pronouncements'. The publication of the report led to widespread criticism. Michael Duggan, the Greater London Council expert on lead wrote in a report to the Council:

If the polarising effect of the Working Party's review is as marked on others as it is on me, then their report will sharpen rather than soften the debate about environmental lead in this country.

His views were notable and these are a few extracts:

They conclude that lead in petrol makes only a minor contribution to children's blood-lead. Their report does include mention of a recent study by Billick and his colleagues in New York which showed a close correlation, over several years, between children's blood-lead and the amount of lead in petrol sold in the area. The Working Party quite rightly point out that correlations do not necessarily mean causality, but the possible 'nothing to do with petrol' explanation advanced in the Report does seem rather strained in comparison with the more obvious one.

The lack of any comprehensive information about blood-lead levels in UK children is at the heart of some of the problems encountered when trying to comment on the effects of environmental lead. The report does give some data from the UK programme carried out to fulfil an EEC Directive, but these are of little help in arriving at any general picture. Probably the most useful data currently available (but not described in the Report) are those from the Birmingham survey carried out in the late 1970's. Of the 429 pre school children examined 15 had blood-lead levels in excess of 35 ug/100 ml – a figure with some status as an 'action level' in the EEC Directive mentioned above. If such a percentage proved to be typical for the UK then it would represent a large number of children. In Greater London for example it would mean that there are about 15,000 children with blood-lead levels in excess of 35 ug/100 ml. One would not think that such a possibility existed from reading the Report. On the basis of the very limited EEC study, the Working Party seemed satisfied that there is no great number of children in the UK with blood-lead levels above 35 ug/100 ml, and that the main cause for concern should be 'hot spots' where only a few people would be exposed.

The Working Party have reviewed most of the studies which have reported on the possible effects of low levels of lead on the intelligence and behaviour of children. . . . The Working Party are critical, with some reason, of all the pre-Needleman studies, but even without Needleman there would be at the very least a strong suspicion that lead produces neuropsychological effects in some children. Why else all the concern over the last decade? However, the Working Party do not seem to share the view that many have held i.e. that prudence demands something less than unequivocal proof of causality before action is taken.

. . . The Working Party describe the testing and assessment of Needleman's high and low lead groups quite fully but some of their criticisms seem unfair. For example, they mentioned that pica was not used as a covariate but do not mention Needleman's reply (published in the open literature) to such a criticism in which he describes further work related to pica, and concludes 'thus pica was not a marker of neurobehavioural deficit'. Again they tend to give an emphasis to blood-lead values which is not in the original work. Needleman's use of tooth-lead rather than blood-lead as a measure of integrated dose is especially valuable in a study of 8/9 year olds whose pre-school exposure would have been more likely than current exposure to cause any damage. For some of the children he gives (almost as an aside) blood-lead data which he had from earlier work, but the whole study is basically reported in terms of tooth-lead. The Working Party then comment 'It is suggested by Needleman that the 4 point mean difference (in IQ) in the two groups is associated with a difference in mean blood-lead concentrations between 23 and 35 ug/100 ml although this is based on blood-lead determinations performed some 4–5 years previously on approximately half of the children involved in the study'. (I imagine Needleman might be surprised at this summary of his work.)

In spite of the prominence given to Needleman's work by the Working Party, their account is unbalanced.

It is dangerously misleading to remark as the Working Party do that 'At present no single blood concentration of lead within this range (35-80 ug/100 ml) can be defined above which an individual child is likely to be harmed'. Leaving aside the error of this statement, if 'harmed' includes interference with haem synthesis, it is true that there are some children in the population who would not suffer any other measurable ill-effects with a blood-lead level up to 80 ug/100 ml. But any regulatory authority must be primarily concerned with the overall occurrence of ill-effects, and who would doubt that if the blood-lead level of our children were distributed within the range 35-80 ug/100 ml there would be a substantial incidence of ill-effects?

The Working Party was set up as a result of concern among both scientists and the public that the petrol-derived lead in our environment may be damaging to the health and development of children. The Working Party have produced a lengthy and detailed report whose major conclusions are that lead in petrol does not make an important contribution to the lead body burden of our child population, and that the blood-lead level of this population is in any case not high enough to give cause for concern.

In reaching the first conclusion the Working Party have concentrated on adult rather than child exposure, and have taken no account of what data there are (from other countries) which suggest marked urban/suburban or urban/rural ratios for children's blood-lead levels. The fallout of petrol-derived airborne lead provides one possible exposure route which could account for these ratios but the Working Party ignore any contribution from lead-in-dust (let alone petrol-derived lead-in-dust) in their apportionment.

In reaching the second conclusion, they assume that the very limited survey carried out in the UK to fulfil the EEC Directive gives a representative picture of levels for pre-school children in the UK. They ignore the broader survey recently made in Birmingham. In contrast to both the EEC and the USEPA they do not believe that the impairment of haem synthesis is an ill-effect. They virtually discount all the epidemiological studies relating to neuropsychological effects made prior to Needleman. And their reservations about his work must be grave indeed, since they have no doubt that there are no deleterious effects on young children at blood-lead levels below 35 ug/100 ml. They even doubt that such effects exist below 80 ug/100 ml.

There are many versions of how the final decision to keep lead in petrol but reduce it to 0.15 grams per litre was taken, but perhaps the most likely was that described by George Brock in *The Times* on May 7, 1982, after a lengthy investigation. He wrote:

The findings show that it was a prolonged barter over tangled priorities and in the end the Ministers went down the line of least expensive resistance. Muddled evidence that the invisible and tasteless lead aerosol emitted by car exhausts may damage children's intelligence was traded with the health and safety of British Leyland and the Government's unwillingness to do anything which costs money about other crucial sources of lead pollution.

Brock reported:

The negotiation began in November 1979 when a working party of civil servants chaired by Mr. John Rowcliffe, a DOE Under Secretary in charge of the Ministry's Central Directorate on Environmental Pollution, started to digest two documents: the Lawther report and a less known but equally important report written by a civil service/industry Committee on the costs and implications of various possible decisions about petrol lead (known by its acronym; WOPLIP report). The working party was to sit for almost 18 months before presenting a divided report before a Cabinet Committee and was attended by, or heard from, the Departments of Health, Transport, Environment, Energy, Industry, The Treasury, and London Transport.
According to a Department of Energy internal memorandum of July 1980 both the DHSS and the DOE began by arguing that not only should there be an immediate cut in the lead content of petrol, but that it should be accompanied by 'a further commitment to lead-free petrol'. 'Some progress has been made' said the note, 'in establishing wider areas of agreement, but it is not possible to resolve the fundamental differences at official level'.

Brock then reported on the findings of the Lawther Committee and the view of Lawther that his report was intended to recommend a reduction in the lead level of petrol to zero. He described the arrival of the Yule and Lansdown preliminary findings and said 'The reports brought back to their department by the DHSS officials present at the meeting created a fear that the Government might announce a cautious cut in lead decision at almost exactly the same moment as a key piece of research advanced knowledge of its dangers.'

Brock continued:

But during that autumn, the push towards the lead-free position was being abandoned. Why?

Two problems were seen as insuperable. No solution to the problem which would really alter lead levels in the atmosphere was going to be cheap, and the dilemma was to settle where the costs should fall. If there is to be a sharp cut but nothing else, the costs fall on the oil companies. If there was to be a gradual phase-out of lead completely, there would be a slightly higher national fuel consumption and the costs would fall on the car manufacturers.

The Department of Industry argued that a move to lead-free petrol ahead of the rest of Europe would weaken British Leyland during the transition. Foreign car manufacturers were better placed to sell cars in Britain running on lead-free, production lines would have to be adapted to make both lead-free and leaded petrol engines and any increase in the cost of cars or fuel might depress demand for cars.

The safety of British Leyland will have found a receptive ear at the E(EA) Cabinet Committee which made the eventual decision . . . to lay the cost on the oil refiners by bringing the lead level down to 0.15 grams per litre by the end of 1985. It was established not to consider ecological questions but micro-industrial problems.

There is little question that Brock was right to assume that it was the position of the car manufacturers that was the key factor, for we know that the petroleum industry had offered lead-free petrol.

The WOPLIP document had reviewed five alternative options for further reducing lead emissions. These were:

Option 1   Install lead filters with a catchment efficiency of 50 per cent on all new vehicles after a certain date;

Option 2   Reduce the lead content of all petrol for all vehicles to 0.15g/l while maintaining the octane quality (as the Federal Republic of Germany has done);

Option 3(1)   Introduce new premium fuel at 95 RON with 0.15g/l lead for new vehicles only while maintaining existing premium and regular petrol with higher lead levels for existing vehicles (until they are substantially phased out in say 10 years time);

Option 3(2)   As in 3(1) but take regular petrol off the market as soon as the new petrol is introduced (these alternatives of Option 3 represent extremes of possible marketing sub-options);

Option 4   Introduce petrol of 92 RON and with a lead level of 0.05-0.08g/l for new vehicles while maintaining existing premium petrol for existing vehicles;

Option 5   Introduce lead-free petrol of 92 RON for new vehicles while maintaining existing premium petrol for existing vehicles.

The Committee tentatively summarised the eventual costs and benefits of these options as follows:

Option	Cost in £m (1978 prices)	Annual total lead emissions expressed as percentages of 1971 total
1 (Lead filters for new vehicles)	70–75 (plus perhaps 4–5 to cover cost of disposal scheme)	50–55
2 (Petrol with unchanged octane quality and 0.15g/l lead for all vehicles)	120–130	35–40
3(1) (95 RON petrol with 0.15g/l lead for new vehicles)	80–85	35–40
3(2) (as at 3(1) but withdrawing existing regular petrol at once)	80–85	35–40
4 (92 RON petrol with 0.05–0.08g/l lead for new vehicles)	200	15–20
5 (92 RON lead-free petrol for new vehicles)	200	0

The Committee did not itself recommend an option on the basis of the data in its report 'because of the need for a more sophisticated medical and scientific evaluation of benefit – and in particular of the value of early benefit'.

It also pointed out that:

it is essential to consider in making a choice whether the option chosen would represent a final solution and not merely be a prelude to further action. The question has to be faced whether if any option other than option five (92 RON lead-free petrol for new vehicles) were chosen, this would prove to be temporary as a result of a subsequent decision to remove lead from petrol altogether. There are substantial cost penalties involved in choosing either option 1 (lead filters for new cars), option 2 (petrol with unchanged octane quality and 0.15 grams per litre of lead for all vehicles), or option 3 (1) or (2) (95 RON petrol with 0.15 grams per litre lead for new vehicles) simply as a prelude to option 5; and the resulting total costs would be very much greater than those of option 5 if pursued in the first instance.

(This emphasis on the fact that lead-free petrol should only be rejected if the decision is likely to have effect for some considerable time fuelled rumours that Whitehall, once the decision to reduce to 0.15 was taken, promised the petroleum industry representatives informally that to compensate them for the costs of modifying refineries, they would 'hold the line' on the decision for at least 10 years.)

The working party commented that in terms of the benefit of reducing lead emissions, option 5 (lead-free) would obviously be the most effective in the long term, but option 2 (reduction to 0.15 grams per litre) would have the advantage of being implementable a year earlier and of having an almost immediate impact by cutting total emission levels to about a third of the 1971 level in 1985. Option 5 would only reduce emissions gradually as older cars disappeared.

CLEAR commissioned the much-respected city firm of management consultants, Coopers and Lybrand Associates, to look at the way decisions had been taken on the issue.

They reported:

> The analysis totally overlooked the further possible option of combining the best elements of options 2 and 5 by (a) stipulating lead-free petrol for new vehicles, and (b) a limit of 0.15 grams per litre for existing vehicles. It is difficult to understand why this alternative option which combines the advantages of options 2 and 5 was not considered by the lead-in-petrol working party. This would still appear to be a practical alternative combining the advantages of (a) as fast as possible reduction in the overall level of lead emissions, (b) the eventual introduction of lead-free petrol, and (c) eliminating uncertainty and giving both the petroleum and motor car industries clearly defined regulations within which to plan.

So it was that on May 11, 1981, Tom King, Minister responsible for 'Environmental Services' rose in the House of Commons to announce what action was to be taken on environmental pollution by lead following the publication of the Lawther report. On the serious problem of old paint, all he announced was that it 'will be tackled by information and advice to local authorities and by increased emphasis on health education programmes'. On leaded water, he made his most positive disclosure – that in cases where drinking water came from lead-lined tanks, and where the only answer was to alter the plumbing, the work would be eligible for home improvement grants.

Then he moved on to lead in petrol:

The Government has decided that maximum permitted lead content of petrol should be reduced as far as is possible, without ruling out the continued use of car engines at present designed – that is, from the present level of 0.40 grams per litre to 0.15 grams per litre. This will reduce by about two-thirds lead emissions from cars ten years earlier than any other practicable method.

Denis Howell, Opposition spokesman, asked:

Is the Minister aware that the Opposition are extremely disappointed on the main issue of principle, namely, lead in petrol? We believe that this is the wrong decision given the two options before the Government of either reducing the maximum to 0.15 grams per litre or going to lead-free petrol immediately. We believe that the latter decision should have been taken now. Is it not inevitable that the environmental and health considerations and the developing public opinion on the subject will make that part of the Government's decision obsolete well before it is implemented? The Opposition will certainly go for lead-free petrol. We believe that it would have been better to give industry and the motorist the necessary time to adjust to that fundamental decision.

He complained about the 'political delay of eighteen months' before the response to Lawther.

The Labour Government reduced the amount of lead in petrol on four occasions. We set up the WOPLIP enquiry that reported in July 1979 and the Lawther working party which reported in March 1980. It is clear from all the leaks over the past year that there has been a departmental dog fight in which the Treasury has routed the DOE and the DHSS. The House itself has not been consulted. . . . Finally, does the Minister agree that the whole of industry would prefer the major decision to be taken now? We shall get the worst of both worlds by reducing the maximum to 0.15 grams per litre in 1985 and then having the further expense of going to a zero level later. The decision is not in the interests of the motor industry or the oil industry and it is certainly not in the interests of future generations of young children. We must therefore register our grave disappointment with it.

Conservative MP, Martin Stevens, asked whether it was true that 'there has been a deal or understanding with the oil industry, namely that in exchange for a level of 0.15 grams there will be no declaration of intent to move to lead-free petrol?'. King denied this.

David Alton, for the Liberals, asked why the Government dismissed the alternative of lead-free petrol he believed had been offered by the petroleum industry.

King replied

It is not merely a question of what the oil companies can do; it is also a question of what cars can use. If there were an immediate move to lead-free petrol as from tomorrow, the vast majority of cars in Britain could not use it. The problem is to achieve the change-over.

If one went down the lead-free route one would have to have a reasonable period of transition.

In answer to another question, King estimated the annual cost of a reduction to 0.15 grams per litre as £200 million. 'For the motorist it will amount to about £25 per year'. His estimate of the increase in petrol prices was about fourpence a gallon.

Howell by now had spotted the point later to be made by Coopers and Lybrand. He asked:

Is it not possible to have a reduction programme simultaneously with the announcement of a lead-free policy to follow it?

On the same day, Lord Bellwin announced the new policy in the House of Lords. 'What it really amounts to is that we are going for most of the loaf now rather than the whole of the loaf later.'

New Scientist commented on May 14:

In choosing a lower limit, the Government has opted for short-term gains. This is a defensible political position. But if the Government thinks that children exposed to less lead than they now are would run no risks, it is sadly mistaken. The best of today's toxicologists agree that there is almost certainly no lower limit below which lead does no harm. Uncomfortable though it may be, this conclusion is crucial. The Government's new limit means that the oil industry will have to invest £400 million to make low lead petrol. In future, the Government – any Government – would, if it wanted further reductions, have a difficult task persuading the industry to invest yet more money before it had recovered this first £400 million. The new limit of lead in petrol could delay, perhaps indefinitely, a total ban.

During the following days all of the spokesmen for the relevant industries declared themselves content with the decision. Everyone concerned with environmental protection declared themselves appalled. The polluters had won the battle. But if they believed the war was over, they were in for a considerable shock.

6.
The CLEAR challenge

WHILE CALIP and others concerned about lead pollution were disappointed by the May 1981 decision not to ban lead in petrol, the decision to reduce to 0.15 grams per litre was a remarkable achievement for those who had sustained a campaign over a number of years with very limited resources of money and manpower. Just the same, it was difficult to see what could now be done. It was at this point that Godfrey Bradman, chairman of a public company, came upon the scene. Bradman at the time lived in Chelsea with his family and read a number of articles about the dangers associated with the heavy traffic passing their home every day. Bradman is an extraordinarily thorough man, and he set out to establish the facts for himself, studying the literature, and meeting a number of the so-called experts, including Professor Patrick Lawther. At first he was reassured by Lawther but as he investigated the issue further he became convinced that the level of risk justified moving house to the fringes of London. Fortunately, Bradman is not a man to look after his own family and remain indifferent to the fate of others. He generously offered the considerable sum of £100,000 to pay for the launch of a fresh campaign. (His contribution did not stop there; his shrewd advice and his constant encouragement were also of great value.) I had myself become concerned about the problem while researching an article for the *Illustrated London News* and, after a meeting with Godfrey Bradman and some of his advisers, accepted an invitation to head up the campaign. We set out to define objectives that, despite our indignation at the attitude of the industries, would be fair and realistic. We were well aware that many influential individuals and organisations had maintained their distance from the anti-lead campaigners for fear of becoming involved in what they cautiously believed could be an over-emotive or unrealistic campaign. To obtain the support we needed we had to be seen to be medically and scientifically sound, and also to be seen to be fair and reasonable about the practical problems of a move to lead-free petrol. It was essential that we asked for what could, in fact, be achieved.

We finally settled for the following five objectives:

1   To urge that the fixed limit of 0.15 grams per litre for lead in petrol should be introduced earlier than the official date of 1985 and be for existing cars only.

2   To demand that as soon as possible, and in any event by early

1985, all new cars sold on the UK market be required to run on lead-free petrol.

3   To demand that as soon as possible, and in any event by early 1985, all petrol stations be required to have lead-free petrol available for sale to the public.

4   To urge that taxation on the sale of petrol should be imposed to create a price advantage to motorists purchasing lead-free petrol.

5   To maintain surveillance on the use of lead generally and to encourage enforcement of any measures necessary to reduce lead pollution wherever it occurs.

In doing this, we accepted the probability that lead would need to be phased out of petrol over a generation of cars, as was being done in the United States, had been done in Japan, and was to be done in Australia.

Outside of CLEAR's inner counsels, Bryce-Smith and others argued that we should demand an immediate ban on lead in petrol for all cars by supporting the introduction of high octane lead-free petrol. The problem was that at that point anyway we simply did not have adequate evidence that high octane lead-free petrol was a realistic possibility. Our objectives, however, did not rule out any particular route to lead-free petrol – high octane, low octane, or an alternative additive – and were, therefore, both fair and flexible.

Let's look at each of the objectives:

To urge that the fixed limit of 0.15 grams per litre for lead in petrol should be introduced earlier than the official date of 1985 and be for existing cars only

This followed the Coopers and Lybrand proposal of a combination of Governmental options – a reduction to 0.15 for existing cars and lead-free petrol for new cars. We explained this at the time as follows:

1 While there is controversy over the extent of modification required and it varies from car to car, we accept that for many vehicles on the road at present some adaptation may be necessary for them to run on unleaded fuel – albeit in some cases of a minor nature. To enforce that adaption could be difficult and unpopular. It would also enable unscrupulous politicians to play on the fears of existing car owners to avoid a move to lead-free. Further, it could call for a considerable input by the car manufacturing and servicing industries and we would prefer that input to be concentrated on the earliest possible introduction of new cars modified to take lead-free petrol.

2   A considerable proportion of cars already on the road will operate on lead-free petrol. One Minister has admitted to a figure of 10%. Some have been manufactured to do so, and others do not require the use of leaded fuel all of the time.

3   Given suitable tax incentives, we believe many existing car owners would voluntarily have their cars adapted to take lead-free petrol and we believe this would be preferable to compulsion.

4   We believe this whole issue of lead in petrol should be looked at afresh without it being necessary for anybody to defend their previous position. Our proposal does not run counter to the Conservative administration's decision to reduce the level to 0.15 grams per litre by 1985, as far as existing cars are concerned (apart from the fact that we believe it should be imposed sooner) but rather calls for an extension of their policy to reduce lead levels. We hope, therefore, this will enable it to approach the public demand for the manufacture of new cars to take unleaded fuel from a less defensive posture than would be the case if its policy had to be completely reversed.

(In fact, the Conservative administration did not respond to this 'olive branch' approach by CLEAR but we still believe it made sense to try and find a positive face-saving solution for Ministers.)

To urge that taxation on the sale of petrol should be imposed to create a price advantage to motorists purchasing lead-free petrol

The aim of this was to make it worthwhile for economy-minded motorists to adapt their existing cars to run on lead-free fuel, and also encourage buyers of new cars to use the unleaded fuel rather than the leaded variety. A high percentage of the money we spend on every gallon of petrol is the tax element and thus it is within the power of the Chancellor of the Exchequer to create suitable incentives.

To demand that as soon as possible, and at any event by early 1985, all new cars sold in the UK market be required to run on lead-free petrol

To demand that as soon as possible, and at any event by early 1985, all petrol stations be required to have lead-free petrol available for sale to the public

It can be seen that CLEAR refrained from taking up a position on the best way to eliminate lead from petrol. There were two reasons for this: first, the issue of how we eliminate lead from petrol was not of importance until after a decision to eliminate lead from petrol. We wanted to concentrate on campaigning on the health issue – our reason for being concerned at all – without becoming embroiled in a complicated dispute over the technicalities of high and low octane. Second, we took the view that until that decision was taken, the industries had a vested interest in emphasising the difficulties and exaggerating the costs; once that decision was taken, however, they had a vested interest in minimising the cost and finding the most efficient way of proceeding to lead-free petrol.

The objectives now fixed, we next had to broaden the base of support. It had been too easy for the industries and politicians to brush off anti-lead campaigners as extreme or fanatical. It was now necessary, armed with sound evidence and our set of objectives, to win as much organisational support as possible. Within nine months CLEAR was supported formally by 17 national organisations, The Advisory Centre for Education, The Association of Directors of Social Services, The Association of Neighbourhood Councils, CALIP, The Association of Community Health Councils for England and Wales, The Cleaner London Campaign, The Conservation Society, Friends of the Earth, The Health Visitors Association, The London Amenity and Transport Association, The Pedestrians Association, The Spastics Society, Transport 2000, The National Children's Centre, The National Union of Teachers, The Ramblers Association and The West Indian Standing Conference. CLEAR thus spoke for a substantial and responsible body of opinion.

We then set up two organisations, the campaigning organisation, to be known as CLEAR, The Campaign for Lead-free Air, with myself as chairman and an Advisory Committee consisting largely of fresh names to the anti-lead movement, many of them experienced directors and workers with other pressure groups who could inject their experience into our planning; and a Charitable Trust, to raise money for research and educational activities, with such distinguished trustees as Dame Elizabeth Ackroyd, former director of the Consumer Council, Sheila Black, journalist and member of the National Consumer Council, Christopher Brasher, Olympic gold medallist and sports writer, Dr. Jonathan Miller, Lord Avebury, then president of the Conservation Society, the Bishop of Birmingham, Christopher Hall, editor of *The Countryman*, Professor Christopher Foster of the management consultants, Coopers and Lybrand, the popular television personality, Dr. David Bellamy, and trade union leader Clive Jenkins.

The next step was to move towards the isolation of the governing party by tying up the opposition. We were able to enlist the support of Liberal leader David Steel, Labour leader, Michael Foot, and SDP Parliamentary leader, Dr. David Owen to endorse the campaign before it was launched. And we then approached

Members of Parliament with our list of objectives, inviting them to sign them as supporters. By the middle of 1982 over 200 MPs had signed the objectives, 35 of them Conservative members. We also had over 50 supporters in the House of Lords.

An office was opened near Kings Cross, my two dedicated colleagues, the Campaign Administrator, Susan Dibb, and the Campaign Assistant, Patricia Simms, were employed, print material was designed, and a launch date fixed for January 25, 1982.

Two men emerged as a source of tremendous strength to CLEAR. One was Bob Stephens to whom I have already referred. The other was the indefatigable Dr. Robin Russell Jones, Senior Registrar at St. John's Hospital in London. Robin had, like Bradman, been convinced by the medical evidence and moved his home out of London. Also like Bradman, he was not satisfied with having reduced the threat to his own children. In addition to a remarkable capacity to accumulate and comprehend medical and scientific information, he is a fluent writer and speaker and became an exceptionally able Deputy Chairman of the campaign. It was a tribute to his grasp of the issue that Professor Michael Rutter was happy to co-edit with him the extended version of the Proceedings of the CLEAR Symposium and to invite Robin and Bob Stephens to contribute the central section of the book on sources of lead exposure.

While we tried to maintain confidentiality in order to make an impact with the launch of CLEAR, it was necessary in order to build up advance support that a considerable number of people knew the plan. One of them turned up at our Kings Cross office and handed me the document that became known as 'the Yellowlees letter'. This was an enormous boost for it was now impossible for our opponents to say there was no high-level support for our claims of a health hazard. We also knew its publication would arouse considerable indignation in the House of Commons where MPs quite rightly do not like to feel that they have been party to decisions without having the benefit of the advice available to Ministers, especially when that advice would appear to have encouraged a different decision from the one the Ministers had taken. It was tempting to employ the letter at the press conference to launch CLEAR, but we felt confident that the press conference would generate adequate publicity on its own and so held the letter back in order to let our opponents waste their gunfire in reply to our launch before striking with what had now become our main weapon. It was, however, to put it mildly, a considerable morale booster to be able to walk into our launch press conference with the letter 'up our sleeves'.

The launch of CLEAR achieved considerable publicity and

immediate support. *The Guardian* in a leading article said:

> When there is such widespread feeling in favour of a reform and a cleaner air bonus at the end of it, the Government can be accused of obstinacy – and worse – in selecting this question as one on which to dig in its heels.

A number of provincial papers published leading articles, all in support of the campaign. Typical was the *South Wales Echo*. It stated:

> We cannot remove the communities from the roads but we can remove the lead from the petrol. It is not sensible to dismiss this pressure group as yet another bunch of highly motivated environmentalists with puritan ideas about technology. The Government must take them seriously.

Less than a fortnight later the Yellowlees letter was published in *The Times*, with a front page news story and an article on the leader pages by myself. I wrote:

> Had the letter been made public at the time it was written, we would now be on our way to lead-free petrol and our CLEAR campaign would never have been necessary.

It is a highly significant letter for three reasons:
● First, while ministers continue to say that there is no convincing evidence that low-level exposure to lead is a real threat to health, their own chief medical officer, Sir Henry Yellowlees, put himself emphatically on the record a year ago that 'there is a strong likelihood that lead in petrol is permanently reducing the IQ of many of our children'. No one can any longer claim that there is no high-level opinion opposed to the use of lead in petrol.

Ministers have to make a choice. They either continue to quote the report of the Lawther committee as evidence that lead in petrol is not the main cause of lead pollution, or they have to accept the advice of their chief medical officer. Yellowlees and Lawther so contradict each other that there is no room for compromise in their views.

● Secondly, those who have up to now criticised the Lawther report have been accused of not being open to reason. That accusation can no longer be made. The letter adds up a a complete rejection of the fundamental approach and conclusions of the Lawther committee.

Lawther's report denied the link between lead in petrol and lead in food.

Sir Henry Yellowlees, on the other hand, says 'lead in petrol is a major contributor to blood-lead acting through the food chain as well as by inhalation'.

● Thirdly, the chief medical officer's letter admits that 'there is no doubt that the simplest and quickest way of reducing general population exposure to lead is by reducing sharply or entirely eliminating lead in petrol'. In this he contradicts ministers who still seek to pinpoint other aspects of lead pollution as the more serious problem.

I find it deeply disturbing, as I believe many MPs will, that such powerfully worded advice should have been restricted to a few permanent secretaries, and possibly to one or two ministers. The use of lead in petrol is an issue of considerable public concern. It is probably the major public health controversy in this country today.

If I am correct in believing that its publication would have caused a public outcry and forced the phasing out of lead in petrol, then its confidentiality contributed to a disastrous decision. We, the taxpayers, employ the chief medical officer, not his Whitehall masters. Do we not have a right to the publication of his advice on such matters before and not after it is watered down or filed away in Whitehall?

The London *Evening Standard* in a leading article that night said: 'The letter specifically knocks on the head Health Minister Kenneth Clarke's argument that more research is needed'. The *Standard* went on:

> Sir Henry's verdict was circulated to a small circle of top civil servants and ministers – though not, of course, to the tax payers who foot the bill or the parents whose children are at risk. Such are the wise ways of Whitehall. Mr. Clarke, presumably, knew all about it. If not, he does now. And, as he says, this Government knows where its duty lies.

The next day *The Times* published a leader stating that the letter 'will, and should, raise the temperature of an already heated issue'. *The Times* went on:

> We should not have to wait until the very last mathematical correlation has been established to announce proudly that there is final proof that children have continued to be blighted while the research was concluded. The balance of risk is clearly such as to justify the maximum control on the emissions of lead poisons.

The Times concluded:

> Society often shies at the cost of eliminating an evil, as it does at the price of stopping the annual slaughter on our roads. But this is not a case of reckless individuals choosing to maim themselves along with others, it concern tens of thousands of children, born and yet to be born, the future generation of this country at risk of being disadvantaged. It is not every child; and the risk is not a certainty. But the risk is too great to bear, and the price of eliminating the poison is far from being too high to pay.

The following day the British Medical Association's Board of Science disclosed its concern:

> On the basis of past scientific evidence, the Board of Science believes that lead taken into the human body is a serious public health hazard. . . . The Board believes that all sources of lead pollution should be eliminated wherever possible.

Professor Thomas Oppe, a paediatrician and former member of the Lawther Committee, was quoted in the newspapers as saying:

> The Board of Science is convinced that low level exposure to lead can be a cause of brain damage. Every effort should be made to reduce lead levels.

On February 10, A. E. J. Yelland, Managing Director of Associated Octel, wrote to *The Times* to say that 'the loudness of the clamour from the CLEAR campaign is not evidence'. He claimed that the media did not provide equal opportunity for opponents of CLEAR and this 'could be described as censorship'. Douglas Harvey of the UK Petroleum Industry Association also wrote to *The Times* to point out that 'the oil industry is now working towards implementing 0.15 grams per litre at considerable expense. Obviously, the major part of this expenditure would be redundant if the Government decided to go to 92-octane unleaded petrol thereafter'.

A Hampstead reader wrote to *The Times:*

> If uncertainty exists, how dare the Government gamble with the health of the country's children, including those of the consumers, who, a Government spokesman says, wish to have high compression engines that require lead in petrol. Surely on consideration they would be prepared to have brighter children and lower-compression engines than risk damage to children, or can their values be so perverse?

In a leader the *Birmingham Post* said:

> Once again it seems that the Government has too readily seized upon the prospect of expense and inconvenience to avoid upsetting noisy and self-interested factions. . . . There is a distressing side-effect of such behaviour in Whitehall and Westminster. The inconsiderate are encouraged to go on poisoning the environment or needlessly destroying until a ridiculously inflated amount of evidence has been gathered against them. Pneumoconiosis in the mining industry, asbestos, by-products of the nuclear industry in bomb testing, pesticides and defoliants, paints and glue, have all claimed countless victims. The cost to the people is too often the one to be counted last. The Government should rid Britain's air of this major potential hazard.

The Guardian reported:

> Certainly the fear of God has been put into Associated Octel, the people who add lead to petrol, who have been showering MPs with documents since CLEAR began work three weeks ago. But their latest manoeuvre, an offer to supply MPs with the Lawther report (which has been available to members free as a public document since it was published in March 1980) has back-fired. Jeff Rooker has put down a motion deploring a private company's bombarding all MPs with offers of a public document, and other members, regardless of party, have been niggled by the high-pressure selling. Octel is meanwhile spending delightfully large sums sending advocates to rival CLEAR's energetic spokesmen all over the country.

Throughout the country local authority leaders and MPs began to announce their support.

On February 20 *The British Medical Journal* published a leader stating:

> The BMJ believes there is a good case for removing lead from petrol: the metal is certainly toxic, and while the worldwide trend is towards lead-free petrol Britain would be wise to follow.

These words are of importance, for despite what follows, the BMJ made clear that it accepted the case for action. It then went on to say – and who would argue with it? – that it believed . . .

> decisions on issues of this kind should be taken on the basis of reliable scientific evidence, not emotional propaganda.

Associated Octel were to frequently quote these last words out of context, implying that the British Medical Journal either had no view on the issue, or opposed a ban on lead in petrol. This was not the case.

Indeed, on May 22, after the CLEAR symposium, the BMJ said:

> Professor Rutter was in no doubt that the evidence was enough to justify Government action to eliminate lead from petrol – *a conclusion shared by the BMJ* and one which we have advocated on general grounds for some time.

After emphasising that further research was needed it said once more:

> Nevertheless, removing lead from petrol will lead to real benefits. Firstly, this action will add to the margin of safety of children living in environments polluted by lead in plumbing, paint, cosmetics or industrial waste. Secondly, if de-leading petrol has similar effects in Britain to those in the United States, average blood-lead concentrations in the community will fall.

The Times returned to the attack with another leading article, this time concentrating on calling for EEC action:

> It is unthinkable that progress should stop short at 1985. It is necessary to ensure that as today's cars grow old, they are superceded by a generation of cars using no lead at all. The right and proper corollary of the Government's policy should have been an announcement that all new cars sold after that date, or the earliest date that the EEC permitted, should run without need of the poison. The sooner an announcement is made to that effect, the better our manufacturers will be able, like their competitors in Japan and America, to start planning for a certainty rather than an uncertainty.

The huge impact of the campaign and the public support that CLEAR had became apparent in March when *The Observer* carried as its front page headline story the results of a public opinion poll CLEAR had commissioned from the MORI organisation. It showed that nine out of ten people in Britain wanted lead banned from petrol.

The sample was a substantial one: 1911 adults, eighteen years of age and older, in 159 constituencies throughout Great Britain. Its results were as follows:

Q1 'As you may know, some of the ingredients in petrol exhaust fumes are harmful. Do you know which particular ingredients these are?'

	%
Carbon monoxide	26
Nitrogen dioxide	0
Water vapour	0
Benzene	0
Lead	70
Carbon dioxide	4
Sulphur dioxide	1
Other	1
Don't know	21

Q2 'Do you think that lead in petrol is a potential health hazard or not? If "yes" do you think it is':

Yes: A very serious health hazard	46	
A fairly serious health hazard	33	91
Or only a slight hazard	12	
No	9	

Q3 'Do you consider that measures to ban lead in petrol are':

Necessary and urgent	55	89
Necessary but not very urgent	34	

Unnecessary 6
Don't know 5

Q4 'Do you think the Government should introduce a law to ensure
that all petrol sold in Britain is lead-free, even if this would put up
petrol prices by a few pence per gallon?'
Yes 77
No 15
Don't know 8

The Observer in its second leader on the subject stated:

> It is hard to think of any other hotly contested political issue on which
> there is such definite public agreement. The poll . . . vindicates the
> campaign's objectives and pays tribute to the skill with which it is
> being conducted. It also puts the Government in a very difficult
> position. Until now Ministers have attempted to batten down the
> hatches and ride out the storm, believing that it would soon blow over.
> They could say, rightly, that they took a major measure against lead
> pollution in last year's decision to cut the amount of the toxic metal
> allowed in petrol by two-thirds. And they have been reluctant to
> appear inconsistent by taking further action and to provoke further
> opposition from the oil and car industries. In their discomfiture, they
> may be tempted to stall a little longer, waiting for further scientific
> evidence to add to the mass that already shows that low levels of lead
> contamination damages children's brains. If they do, they will forfeit
> such respect as their present position still enjoys . . .

> The one substantial question for the Government to resolve is whether
> society is prepared to accept some inconvenience to the car industry
> and a few more pence on the price of a gallon of petrol to protect its
> children. After today's poll there can be no further doubt that it is,
> and the Government should hesitate no longer.

The Guardian published a leader the following day stating that an
EEC-wide ban should be a priority on which the Government might
usefully give a lead:

> Failing such an agreement, the Government will have to take unilateral
> action even if this means effectively barring the import of some of its
> partners' vehicles.

The Daily Telegraph reported that the Government was 'losing the
lead argument'. A follow-up poll of general practitioners by *Doctor*
magazine revealed that 60% believed that 'atmospheric lead even in
small quantities is harmful' and 62% wanted an immediate ban on
lead in petrol.

CLEAR had planned a reduction in the momentum of its

campaign during March and April prior to the big international symposium planned for May. No campaign can on its own sustain a high level of public attention throughout the year. However, CLEAR had an unexpected ally in Associated Octel's executives and trade unionists who launched a letter-writing campaign to newspapers. Inevitably, we had to reply to the letters. The result was that the issue maintained its visibility to a greater extent than we had hoped. (Associated Octel were to make the same mistake even more expensively later in the year when they spent at least £100,000 on a national newspaper advertising campaign. Not only was CLEAR able to achieve equal prominence at no expense by writing letters in response to these ads, but they provoked considerable correspondence by outraged members of the public. CLEAR found itself hoping that Associated Octel would continue its campaign). Perhaps the flavour of the 'letters to the editor' debate is best conveyed by a series of letters that appeared in the *Financial Times*. (I have edited them slightly for space reasons only):

The Argument about Lead-free Air
From the Secretary, Transport and General Workers' Union Shift Branch, Associated Octel, 15 March 1982

Sir. – The activities of CLEAR – the Campaign for Lead-free Air – have been receiving a lot of publicity recently. I am the secretary of the TGWU Shift Branch at Associated Octel, the company which manufactures lead additives for petrol.

I speak on behalf of all our members when I say that I am seriously disturbed by the allegations being made by the campaigners and in particular by Des Wilson, their chairman. A lot of their statements are misleading in the extreme. We fully support Octel in the steps it is taking to present the true facts of the case.

CLEAR claims that other countries, such as the US and Japan, have banned leaded petrol or are phasing it out on health grounds. This is not true. There is no country in the world which has introduced such a ban. In the US as much leaded fuel is sold as unleaded and the reason they introduced lead-free petrol in the first place was nothing to do with health. It was because of smog problems caused by climatic conditions not experienced in the UK.

CLEAR claims that Associated Octel is not a responsible company. Octel has an excellent safety record and has made a major contribution to health and safety within the lead industry. . . .

CLEAR claims that there is new evidence linking children's intelligence with lead levels. This is a palpable untruth. Research is still going on to establish the true facts of the matter. But experts have not found a shred of evidence to prove that lead in petrol is poisoning children's brains.

Does Des Wilson think that any of us would work for Octel if the company was poisoning our children? There is no way it could pay us enough to jeopardise our own children's health or anyone else's.

Mr. Wilson is not a doctor, a scientific researcher or an expert on the properties of lead. He is, though, a gifted speaker and a man who, by trading on people's emotions, is capable of influencing others.

What would be the result for this country if Mr. Wilson was successful in swaying public opinion? The abolition of lead would cost more than £450m every year. Jobs would be lost, cars would be less efficient and all to no effect.

It isn't only Octel which makes these points. Many eminent people support the use of lead in petrol. One person in particular is Dr. Barltrop who says: 'It is difficult to understand why so much attention has been given to less significant sources such as lead in gasoline, the abolition of which would not alter the incidence of lead poisoning at all'. I think it is significant that Dr. Barltrop is director of the department of child health at Westminster Children's Hospital, London.

G. Stokes

Reducing Lead Intake: Many Fumes that Pollute
From Mr. G. Oxley, 26 March 1982
Sir. – As an employee of Associated Octel. . . .

I am bound to be accused of having a vested interest in retaining lead in petrol but, as a scientist educated and trained in critical judgment, I feel I must point out a fundamental fallacy in the arguments of the anti-lead lobby. This lobby builds its case on the evidence in published scientific work which suggests an association between blood-lead values, lead content of children's milk-teeth, etc., and factors such as IQ and hyperactivity. At best, these associations are very poorly defined but leaving that aside, this still does not establish a cause and effect relationship.

In the case of lead burden association with IQ or hyperactivity, surely the underlying cause is poor social conditions. Old and dilapidated housing, poor diet and general deprivation are the conditions for higher than normal lead intake from water, food, old lead-based paint, etc. They are equally the conditions which are highly likely to retard a child's mental development and create stress within the family group.

I must admit to a genuine respect for Mr. Des Wilson when he was conducting the 'Shelter' campaign. If he is now concerned to see lead intake reduced and children's development opportunities improved, he should campaign for better social conditions and not allow himself to be persuaded by the facile arguments of those campaigning against lead in petrol. In short, there are better ways of spending available resources.

G. R. Oxley

The Argument about Lead-free Air
From Dr. R. Russell Jones, 23 March 1982

Sir. – I have no reason to doubt the sincerity of Mr. Stokes' letter but its contents reveal that he has been seriously misinformed on virtually every aspect of the lead-in-petrol issue.

He states that legislation banning the use of lead additives in the United States was 'nothing to do with health'. I quote from a United States federal document published in 1973, two years prior to the introduction of lead-free gasoline. 'The scheduled reduction in the use of lead additives in gasoline to achieve a significant reduction in lead emissions from motor vehicles by 1978, is based on the finding that lead particle emissions from motor vehicles present a significant risk of harm to the health of urban populations, particularly the health of city children. . . .' It should be remembered that the Ethyl Corporation took the Environmental Protection Agency to the Court of Appeal in an unsuccessful attempt to frustrate legislation controlling lead emissions into the atmosphere. The Court ruled that lead emissions from motor vehicles did constitute a significant risk of harm to the health of urban children.

Mr. Stokes' second statement is that there is no new evidence linking children's intelligence with lead levels. Since the DHSS working party published its report 'Lead and health' in 1980, four major papers have appeared in the scientific literature which have a direct bearing on the debate: *inter alia*, they have shown lead levels can be predicted on the basis of EEG (electroencephalographic) recordings in normal children; effects on brain-wave potentials down to blood-lead levels of seven micrograms/decilitre in pre-school children (the bottom end of the normal range); a seven-point IQ deficit in London school children around a mean blood level of 13.52

micrograms per decilitre; and a significant association between lead burden and the proportion of time that children concentrate while in the classroom. This list is by no means comprehensive.

His third statement that, 'experts have not found a shred of evidence to prove that lead in petrol is poisoning children's brains', betrays a similar ignorance of the scientific literature. From 1970–76 the US Government monitored the lead levels of 178,000 New York school children, and established a direct correlation between mean blood lead levels and the amount of leaded gasoline sold in the New York area during that same period. It is certainly true, as Dr. Barltrop says, that removing lead in petrol would not abolish the incidence of symptomatic lead poisoning. But this observation ignores the growing realisation that low level lead exposure is a major cause of intellectual deficit and behavioural disorders in urban children. These deleterious effects are now so prevalent that they have come to be regarded as typical, but the health effects of lead in petrol are nothing less than catastrophic when applied to the population as a whole. . . .

Dr. Robin Russell Jones

From Mr. W. McMillan, 26 March 1982
Sir. – It is unfortunate that in his letter Dr. Robin Russell Jones appeared to impugn the scientific integrity of professional people in the employ of Associated Octel and suggest that those of us with trade union backgrounds have been misinformed. . . .

It is axiomatic that a campaign concerning itself with air pollution will examine the whole problem. Every major city in the UK has allowed efficient pollution-free electric tramcars to be replaced by diesel 'buses with their noxious, polluting (and non lead) exhaust fumes and is permitting ever-larger diesel lorries to use wider roads within their boundaries.

Toxic fumes from millions of gas fires and central heating boilers are allowed to pour into the air we breath, yet CLEAR and its supporters raise not a word of complaint.

For over 10 years Associated Octel, deeply concerned that our wasteful use of carboniferous fuel was a threat to the quality of life for future generations, has, in common with the oil and motor industries, been engaged in the development of filter technology and high efficiency engines. . . .

The difference between CLEAR campaigners and those of us who work in the petrochemical industry is that, while claiming no monopoly of truth and virtue, we work with our professional and medical management towards a cleaner environment and a more responsible attitude towards the conservation of finite materials, CLEAR clings tenaciously to a single issue. Its genuine doubts and fears seem to have blinded it to the fact that we have common cause in our wish to make the world a better place for us all to share.

Wallace E. McMillan

The Continuing Argument about Lead in Petrol
From the Chief Medical Officer, Associated Octel Co, 31 March 1982

Sir. – Dr. Jones (March 23) maintains that Mr. Stokes was misinformed in his letter of March 15 on the matter of the use of lead-free petrol in the US. This is not so. The reason why lead-free petrol had to be made available was because of the introduction of a noble metal catalyst incorporated into the exhaust system to reduce gaseous emissions held responsible for the formation of photo-chemical smog in California, Los Angeles in particular. The presence of lead inactivated the catalyst. Had the catalyst not been required the use of lead additives in petrol would have been reduced, but not eliminated. At the present time about half the cars in the US are catalyst equipped and require lead-free petrol, but the older cars with no catalysts still run on leaded petrol of greater lead content than is permissible in EEC countries.

The present debate in the US is whether or not to continue with the lead phasedown programme as they are already in the area of diminishing returns. There is no evidence from the US that the use of lead-free petrol has improved the health of the nation by a reduction of lead absorption and consideration is being given to a possible extension of the use of leaded petrol. The studies in Frankfurt, Germany of blood-lead concentrations in the city population after lead in petrol had been reduced from 0.4 g/l to 0.15 g/l in 1976, confirmed the minimal effect of such action.

The new evidence quoted by Dr. Jones linking chidren's intelligence with lead levels is no more confirmatory of adverse effects than earlier studies. It is interesting how Dr. Jones appears studiously to avoid mentioning those studies which have shown no effects at concentrations of lead in blood considerably in excess of those quoted by him.

His interpretation of the study of New York school children is fallacious. No correlation was shown between blood-lead and leaded petrol sold in New York; the data given related to petrol sold in the area around New York, which differed from that sold in the city. There was, however, a correlation between a reduction in blood-lead levels and improvement in home conditions, as a result of elimination, or reduction, of household lead-based paint. Also, as the blood-lead screening programme progressed, children were included from areas of lower risk, who would be expected to have lower concentrations of lead in their blood.

There is no evidence which shows 'that low level lead exposure is a major cause of intellectual deficit in urban children' or that 'the health effects of lead in petrol are nothing less than catastrophic, when applied to the population as a whole'. Such emotive language is inexcusable in an accredited professional. Lead in petrol makes a small contribution to the body burden of lead, estimated by measurement as about 10 per cent, as shown by the Frankfurt study.

During the 1970s, the amount of lead used in petrol in the UK remained much the same annually, but lead in food decreased, as shown by surveys of the Ministry of Agriculture and Fisheries, as also did lead in blood (shown by the EEC survey). These findings do not indicate a significant level of contribution from lead in petrol to the body burden and lend no support to the exaggerated claims of the Campaign for Lead-Free Air, as expressed by Dr. Jones.

Dr. P. S. I. Barry

The Argument about Lead in Petrol
From Dr. R. Russell Jones, 2 April 1982

Sir. – Dr. Barry chastises me for 'studiously avoiding' negative studies . . . that is studies which have failed to establish a relationship between increased lead burden and reduced intelligence in children.

There are few such studies in the literature but none is particularly recent and none involved surveys of the general population. Subjects were selected usually on the basis of their proximity to a local source of pollution, such as a lead smelter, or a battery factory, and compared with other children from the same area. The fact that these other children would also have been highly contaminated prevents any useful conclusions being drawn. What is certain is that no study has ever shown lead to have any beneficial effects in children, and surveys which involve unselected groups have invariably demonstrated a correlation between increased lead burden and intellectual deficit.

The second area where Dr. Barry is in error is when he states that 'There is no evidence from the US that the use of lead-free petrol has improved the health of the nation by a reduction of lead absorption.' The Centre for Diseases Control in America has just released a document demonstrating that a 55% reduction in the amount of lead used at refineries over the period 1976–80 was paralleled by a 36%

reduction in the lead level of American children. This nationwide survey confirms the findings of the New York study (which was disputed by Dr. Barry in his letter) and is of far greater relevance than the Frankfurt study, which was carried out on adults and not children. As a direct consequence of this new information, it has been reported that the US Environmental Protection Agency has now decided to drop any plans it may have had to relax legislation controlling lead emissions from motor vehicles.

Dr. Robin Russell Jones

The Argument about Lead in Petrol
From the Chairman, Campaign for Lead-free Air, 2 April 1982

Sir. – You have now published four letters from Associated Octel employees attacking CLEAR's campaign to eliminate lead from petrol. While CLEAR is motivated by concern about the health risk to children, Associated Octel exists to make a profit. We have no philosophical objection to profit – our concern arises when it is achieved at the expense of public health. While we would dispute nearly every detail and opinion in the letters, I will answer them generally.

They brush aside the medical evidence in such fashion that they discredit themselves. Even the authorities in this country accept the health risk; that is why they recently decided to reduce lead in petrol substantially. In other countries it is being phased out altogether, as much because of the health risk from lead as to protect catalytic converters introduced to control other emissions.

The Associated Octel defensive letter-writing campaign cannot obscure the central facts: that lead is a brain poison; it is emitted from car exhausts at the rate of 10,000 tonnes per year; it is absorbed into the body from the air; it can also be absorbed into the body via food; children are more susceptible to its ill effects than adults; lead levels in inner city areas are much greater than in rural areas because of the heavier traffic; and that there is a series of reports that link lead in petrol with reduced intelligence in children, hyperactivity, low concentration and behavioural problems.

It cannot be said often enough that the harm to children may never be proved conclusively; the issue at stake is whether the probability of risk has been established. In our view it has been. No one denies that lead can be eliminated from petrol and the only issue at stake is the cost. The importance of the recently-published poll by a reputable company is that it showed that nearly 8 out of 10 people were prepared to pay that price. The technical answers are there, and the public will is there, and the desire of one company to protect its profits cannot be allowed to stand in the way of change.

Des Wilson

In May the Labour Party NEC announced that it would include the introduction of lead-free petrol as a top priority in the next election manifesto. The NEC said that it would . . .

require in law that at the earliest possible date all new cars sold in Britain must be made to run on lead-free petrol; ensure that all petrol stations must have lead-free petrol available for sale; phase out over a generation of cars the use of lead in petrol; impose taxation on the sale of petrol to create a price advantage to the motorist purchasing lead-free petrol.

Shortly afterwards the CLEAR symposium took place and each day the media carried reports of the various papers presented. The conclusions of Professor Rutter were widely reported.

Geoffrey Lean, *The Observer's* outstanding writer on environmental matters, who has himself made a tremendous contribution on this issue by his well-informed and committed reporting of it over the years, wrote in *The Observer* the following Sunday that:

Last week's call by Professor Michael Rutter, one of the world's leading child psychiatrists, has made a strong impact. Professor Rutter is a member of the Committee most respected in Whitehall and officials have frequently pointed to his signature on the Lawther report as showing that there is no need for a ban. His statement signals that the weight of medical opinion has now moved behind a ban. This is the result of a bold gamble by CLEAR. . . . It invited Professor Rutter to chair the symposium, not knowing whether he had changed his mind since signing the Lawther report, but confident that he would make up his mind on the evidence. To experts in the audience the meeting took on the atmosphere of a tribunal rather than a symposium, with Professor Rutter keenly questioning each speaker. By the end of the three day conference most were expecting a cautious and qualified endorsement of lead-free fuel. But after a thoughtful 5,000 word review of the evidence, Professor Rutter called trenchantly and unequivocally for immediate action.

He described the reduction announced by the Government last year as an unacceptable compromise without clear advantages and with definite disadvantages. He added: 'The evidence suggests that the removal of lead from petrol would have a quite substantial effect in reducing lead pollution, and the costs are quite modest by any reasonable standard.'

In passing he demolished many of the basic arguments of the Lawther Committee's report. . . . His statement demolishes the entire platform on which the Government has stood. And, even worse for Ministers, it is not an isolated event. A substantial number of the Lawther Committee's members have now come to similar conclusions.

The Committee has split into hard-line opponents of a ban, many of whom failed even to reply to invitations to the symposium, and others who are moved towards recommending a ban. Five of the 12 members attended the meeting.

J. E. Winterbottom, Chief Executive of the Associated Octel Company, showed his contempt for Rutter's reputation by writing to the *Liverpool Daily Post*:

> It would indeed be surprising if the Chairman of a three-day international conference which was sponsored by CLEAR whose avowed intention is to remove lead from petrol had come up with any other conclusion than that you report. . . . Indeed, had he done otherwise we could well have expected the organisers to ask for their money back.

Support for CLEAR began to achieve avalanche proportions. Later in May the Inner London Education Authority came out firmly for a ban on lead in petrol. It decided to ask other local authorities to join in an approach to Government:

> We do not find it acceptable that serious risks can be tolerated in this country on economic grounds when several other major industrial nations have opted for lead-free petrol or for petrol with a very low lead level when confronted with the same problem.

The Government twice refused ILEA a meeting.

The National Society for Clean Air, the environmental organisation which has influence with both industry and local authority environmental officers, decided to 'support the ultimate objection of lead-free petrol' and declared that 'this should be mandatory for all new cars at the earliest opportunity'. This decision was significant for two reasons. Firstly, the Society had considerable involvement from petroleum companies. Secondly, Lawther had been a major figure in the Society for many years and was a former President. The Society had thus effectively over-ruled the financial vested interests of the former and the scientific opinions of the latter. In its magazine *Clean Air* it said its policy reflected its primary concern for clean air 'and the decision of the Council that the elimination of lead in petrol is justified to control one route by which lead reaches the human body.'

The Institution of Environmental Health Officers, representing local authority environmental health officers all over the country, sent evidence to the Royal Commission on Environmental Pollution that . . .

> whilst the Government's attitude to a reduction of the lead content of petrol to 0.15 grams per litre is acceptable in the short-term . . . the Government must also give a time when petrol will be lead-free and new cars will be required to function on lead-free petrol.

This was also of considerable significance, for environmental health officers represent a considerable body of experience and knowledge on environmental pollution and also the level of public concern at local level. The Institution had until then remained cautious on the seriousness of petrol-lead pollution. It informed the Commission that whilst the final deadline would be based on cost and economics . . .

> if we were to wait for the economic situation to be right for any pollution control scheme then it is unlikely we would ever achieve an improvement in the environment.

The National Association of Health Authorities in England and Wales decided at its AGM to call upon the Secretary of State for Health and Social Services 'to make a firm commitment to the aims of CLEAR by putting pressure on his cabinet colleagues to bring about a speedy and progressive removal of lead additives in petrol and other sources of lead pollution.' The National Association of Youth Clubs, at its annual conference passed a resolution calling for lead-free petrol, as did the National Association of Head Teachers at its national conference. It stated, 'We consider that this substance should be eliminated, bearing in mind the available medical evidence concerning its effect upon behaviour, health and intelligence of the children we teach.' It obtained further support from the National Union of Teachers, with the Maternity Alliance, a national organisation concerned with the problems of mothers and babies, announced that 'lead in petrol should immediately be banned and replaced with safer additives'.

Alf Dubs, Member of Parliament for Battersea South, introduced under the Ten Minute Rule a Bill in the House of Commons calling for the compulsory sale of lead-free petrol. The first reading was unopposed, although Dubs accepted that it would fail in the end for lack of Parliamentary time.

Dubs told the House: '. . . there are no vested interests arguing to take lead out of petrol. Our view is based simply on the need to safeguard the health and well-being of children. Vested interests seek to oppose the measures.' He said that there was 'massive support in my constituency for the measure. . . . The Lawther report is rapidly on the way to being utterly discredited.'

The Scottish National Party leader in the House of Commons, Donald Stewart, MP, wrote to CLEAR to say:

> In our present state of knowledge of the damage that is being done to children, we give our full support to the campaign for the removal of all lead from petrol as soon as possible. We have been aware of the damaging and detrimental effect of high blood-lead levels for some time in Scotland, as we also have a serious problem with lead in the water supply because of lead plumbing. High lead levels in the air are worsening an already worrying problem in Scotland.

In June 1982 the BBC broadcast a 45 minute report on Radio 4 by its science contributor, James Wilkinson. It was in this programme that Dr. William Yule of the Lawther Committee acknowledged 'It would be prudent to remove lead from petrol', but he emphasised 'that is a personal opinion, and it is not an opinion that comes about on the readings of the scientific literature. There just isn't evidence around to come to that conclusion.' Dr. Richard Lansdown, also on the Lawther Committee said:

> I think I have become less sceptical about the potential risks of moderate levels of lead between 12 and 40 or 50. In 1974 some colleagues and I published a paper in *The Lancet* in which we suggested that children with moderately raised levels of lead were not at risk. Now I think I would regard that view with some scepticism and I would say that perhaps there is a greater danger than I hitherto thought. I think that we should consider revising downwards the previously accepted safe level, but I would stress that we should consider it. I don't think we yet have enough information to be certain on this.

While these cautious remarks were helpful there were some particularly strange contributions by Lawther.

In one he said:

> You don't take half a cup of blood from a child or an adult. In many of the experiments you take one drop and then you put that on filter paper and you cut out a little circle of that and then flash it in a special machine. And I think that – it might appear facetious – but I think that a fly with dirty feet walking over that particular specimen could alter it very considerably, and of course it makes cleaning the skin so important. If a child has dirty skin or anything, you have whacking great bits of lead in it. So it is very difficult.

No-one has so far been able to understand what that meant.

Even more strange was a later Lawther contribution. He

admitted that he would like to see lead out of petrol, water, and food but added:

> I must say in all fairness that my reading of the literature on the absorption of lead from various sources does not lead me to believe that there will be a dramatic decrease following the reduction. There will be a very welcome decrease, but I wouldn't think that we are necessarily all going to have virtually zero blood-leads following this, however welcome it might be.

As no-one had ever suggested that we would end up with zero, this contribution also remained inexplicable.

The programme also contained a passage from Bob Everett from General Motors in the United States who said of the move to unleaded fuel there:

> Looking back I don't think that the technical challenge was nearly as significant as the technical challenge to meet other emission standards . . . there are some pluses that go along without lead that you have also to consider. Lead can contaminate the oil, does contaminate the oil more so than unleaded . . . lead obviously fouls spark plugs. Without lead we can very comfortably run many of our cars 30–50,000 miles or more without a spark plug change. These are expenses that the consumer no longer has to bear. Just the operating on leaded or unleaded as far as the engine performance and so forth is not a very difficult technical obstacle.

Another point to emerge out of the programme was the difficulty that Octel may have even convincing the car manufacturers that they should employ their filter. Ron Mellers of Ford said:

> It is undoubtedly true that you can remove some lead from exhaust gases and one of the major commercial suppliers of lead additives (Octel) have done considerable work in this field. . . . The filters work much better under light driving round town conditions and do have a tendency to blow lead into the air when you accelerate out of the urban environment and on to the motorway. Also on high speed runs the filter efficiency is considerably less. Filters are bulky, difficult to fit to existing cars, costly, and would require replacing at regular intervals.

On September 9, CLEAR launched its autumn campaign. The most noticeable feature of the press conference was a contribution by Gerald Kaufman, Shadow Cabinet Environmental spokesman, who irrevocably committed Labour to a ban on lead. Ministers, he said, 'can no longer prevaricate . . . the sooner proper notice is given to industry, the cheaper the whole exercise becomes. . . . Appropriate tax concessions should be made to assist in the transition period.'

He stated:

> I confirm that the next Labour Government will abolish all lead in petrol and we look to the motor industry to be planning now for that eventuality.

At the same press conference Robin Russell Jones unveiled a CLEAR survey of local authorities. It showed that 85 per cent of local authorities that had taken a policy decision on lead in petrol supported the drive to have it eliminated. Russell Jones said:

> We believe that extensive local authority support for a ban on lead in petrol partly reflects their feeling of impotence in the face of levels in air and dust in their areas. Having undertaken monitoring and established that the problem of environmental lead is a serious one, local authorities are frustrated to discover that they are unable to take any local action to protect the people in their area because the main source of lead pollution is emissions from car exhausts.

Kaufman's appearance at the CLEAR press conference signalled the start of a spectacular political season for CLEAR. The following week the Trades Union Congress overwhelmingly passed a resolution moved by Bill Sirs of the Iron and Steel Trades Confederation calling for a ban on lead in petrol. The Liberal Party's Assembly unanimously passed a resolution calling for a ban on lead in petrol within five years, and two weeks later, the Social Democratic Party made lead-free petrol part of its preventative health policy.

Thus the Conservatives have become isolated as the only political party in Britain still supporting the addition of lead to petrol.

After six months of the CLEAR campaign the two sides in the dispute could be lined up as follows:

Supporting lead in petrol	*Calling for a ban on lead in petrol*
DOE Minister Giles Shaw and his civil servants	The Labour Party
	The Liberal Party
Health Minister Kenneth Clarke and his civil servants	The Social Democratic Party
	The Scottish National Party
Transport Minister Lynda Chalker and her civil servants	The Ecology Party
	Over 100 local authorities
The petroleum industry	The National Consumer Council
The car manufacturers	The Consumer's Association
The lead industry	The National Society for Clean Air
Associated Octel	The Institution of Environmental Health Officers

Supporting lead in petrol	*Calling for a ban on lead in petrol*
	The Trades Union Congress (representing 11 million trade unionists)
	The National Association of Health Authorities
	The National Association of Head Teachers
	The Inner London Education Authority
	The National Association of Youth Clubs
	The National Association of Women's Clubs
	The Advisory Centre for Education
	The Association of Directors of Social Services
	The Association of Neighbourhood Councils
	CALIP
	The Association of Community Health Councils for England and Wales
	The Cleaner London Campaign
	The Conservation Society
	Friends of the Earth
	The Health Visitors Association
	The London Amenity and Transport Association
	The Pedestrians Association
	The Spastics Society
	Transport 2000
	The National Children's Centre
	The Rambler's Association
	The West Indian Standing Conference
	200 Members of Parliament
	Over 50 Members of the House of Lords
	60% of GPs (*Doctor* magazine poll)
	90% of British public (MORI poll)

Supporting lead in petrol	*Calling for a ban on lead in petrol*
	The Times
	The Observer
	The Guardian
	The London Evening Standard
	Doctor magazine
	World Medicine
	New Scientist
	The British Medical Journal

This support for CLEAR did not arise as a result of one-sided propaganda. On the contrary, the Government had used all of its considerable authority and communications power to defend its position. Associated Octel had spent a small fortune circulating nearly all of the organisations considering the matters, every local authority in the country, every Member of Parliament and the media.

Still, as the end of 1982 approached, Ministers remained obstinate, guyed up by their equally stubborn advisers and the support of the financial vested interests.

Royal commission . . . on lead or whitewash?

The Royal Commission on Environmental Pollution was established in 1970 and while it has produced a number of reports on air pollution control, nuclear power, agriculture and pollution, oil pollution of the sea, etc, it would be an exaggeration to say that it has become a power in the land. For instance, by December 8, 1981, it had still not received a Government response to its January 1976 report on air pollution control. Its chairman is Professor T. R. E. Southwood, whose background is zoology and its 16 members include F. G. Larmanie, General Manager of British Petroleum's Environmental Control Centre and a former General Manager of its Public Affairs and Information Section, a section which had in the past played down the health risk of lead in petrol. Another is Professor Barbara Clayton, Lawther Committee member and well-known sceptic on the health effects of lead in petrol. In March 1982, after the launch of CLEAR, this Commission announced that it was to enquire into the 'environmental aspects of lead pollution'. It said it would enquire into four issues:

1 The sources of environmental lead pollution and pathways to man, in particular quantitative data having a bearing on the relative significance of different sources and pathways to the body burden in man.

2 Methods of reducing lead in the environment and human uptake.
3 Technical and economic implications of different options, and their environmental effects, for further reducing or eliminating lead from petrol.
4 Lead pollution and wildlife.

What was astonishing was the exclusion of an enquiry into the health hazard of lead in petrol. Its defence for this was:

> The Commission recognises that the possible effects of low levels of lead pollution on human health and behaviour are a difficult subject of great importance. In view of the several recent evaluations of data on the subject [presumably this meant the Lawther report], and the continuing research, the Commission does not feel it would be sensible at this time to undertake a fresh evaluation of the evidence in this field.

This was clearly disastrous, and CLEAR submitted evidence challenging the Commission's self-imposed limitations:

> In establishing its objectives, the Commission hopes to avoid covering similar territory covered by the DHSS working party chaired by Professor Patrick Lawther, yet that Committee's report itself is sufficiently controversial to demand a full re-evaluation of the evidence it considered. Furthermore, substantial new evidence has accumulated since the Lawther Committee reported. This new evidence concerns both the contribution from lead in petrol to body lead burdens and the health effects.
> For the Commission to give higher priority at this point to technical and economic implications of the elimination of lead from petrol than it intends to give to the environmental hazard that lead in petrol causes, suggests a failure to appreciate both the urgent need for a fresh examination of the hazard, or the widespread concern throughout the country on this issue. The Commission's present objectives put it in danger of approaching the matter on industry's terms, and this cannot be acceptable.
> The Commission should also consider a further problem. Ministers are, on the lead issue, already stating (in the words of one), 'We shall of course take into account any recommendations made to us by the Royal Commission on Environmental Pollution'. Thus the Commission is in danger as being cast in the familiar role of such Commissions – as a way whereby Ministers can postpone or avoid acting on public concern. If the Commission reports without including a review of the health question, its report will be open to serious misrepresentation by Ministers who wish to maintain the status quo. It will not be adequate for the Commission to say that it did not look into the question; ordinary members of the public, who will not see the Commission's report, or be able to follow all the subtleties of the debate, will assume

– in our view, logically assume – that the Commission has looked into this area. Thus we can foresee already the claim that 'the Royal Commission did not reinforce the case that there is a health hazard' being made by those whose record has been, so far, to distort all the available evidence and information on the issue. The effect of declining to review the health evidence, therefore, will be that the Commission will inadvertently have enabled the pro-lead lobby to create the impression that the Commission has reviewed it and rejected it.

In our view the Commission cannot adequately approach the task it has set itself without beginning with the fundamental question: Do we *need* to eliminate lead from petrol? That question is only partly answered by an investigation of sources of exposure; it can only be fully answered by examination of the evidence related to its effect on human health and behaviour.

For these reasons we urge the Commission to widen its brief to cover the health aspects: failure to do so will make its work virtually irrelevant.

While the Commission sought later to suggest that it would at least in part cover the health question, it was significant that the DHSS, when asked by myself to supply a copy of its evidence to the Royal Commission, replied:

As the Royal Commission has not invited evidence on the possible effects of lead on health, DHSS has not submitted separate departmental evidence.

In its evidence, CLEAR emphasised the importance of the elimination of lead from petrol as 'the one step that the authorities can take that will reduce a substantial area of lead pollution (1) efficiently, (2) permanently, and (3) to the benefit of the nation as a whole – this one act will create a margin of safety for everyone, irrespective of other sources of lead pollution they face.' CLEAR's evidence argued that Lawther was both discredited and out-dated, challenged the claim by Ministers that they were taking the most effective action on lead in petrol, argued that the Commission must take a decision based on the risk factor involved, and demonstrated at considerable length the strength of the evidence of health hazard and the source of lead pollution.

Our evidence concluded:

The fact of the matter is that the structure of the British administrative and political system is such that it is made for compromise. A number of different Ministers have been involved in the decision on lead in petrol and much of their dialogue has been with the industries concerned. This is why it is vital that the Commission look at this matter, as its title suggests it should, from an *environmental* point of view alone and should firmly state whether or not in *environmental* terms lead in petrol makes sense or not. We cannot believe that the Commission could say that it does.

Given the controversial nature of this issue, the power of the financial vested interest in favour of the status quo and the imperative for the Government to maintain its present position for political reasons if it possibly can, the Commission in looking into this issue undertakes a considerable responsibility. It should not allow itself to forget that it is a Royal Commission into *Environmental Pollution*, not the economics or technical problems of the motor car industry or the petroleum industry.

On July 2, 1982, I went with Robin Russell Jones and Robert Stephens to meet the full Commission. I quote from the minutes of the meeting:

> Mr. Wilson said . . . the Commission should consider the evidence for health effects of exposure to low levels of lead. The public concern was not about pathways of lead or about technological and economic issues, but about whether lead was a threat to children. If environmental levels of lead did not present a health threat it was pointless to debate the other questions. Either the Commission was already convinced of a risk to health, or it had to consider the evidence . . . the public was looking for objective guidance from a body such as the Commission in an area of genuine scientific controversy.

We were listened to with the courtesy that one would expect on these occasions. It was noticeable that whilst we reviewed the health evidence, Professor Barbara Clayton made no attempt to ask a question or indicate areas where she would need to be convinced (Professor Clayton rarely takes part in the public debate and this makes it extremely difficult to identify her justifications for a negative position on the issue, let alone to undertake any dialogue with her.)

Later I wrote to the secretary to the Commission to enquire whether they had reconsidered their decision to look into the health issue; I was told:

> As can be demonstrated from its previous reports, the Commission has a track record of flexibility and a willingness to redefine its terms of reference for a study as its investigations proceed.

There is, however, no evidence that the DHSS has subsequently been asked to give evidence on the health issue. In the circumstances, I felt it necessary to remind CLEAR supporters in the campaign newspaper that all Royal Commissions had a 'track record' of 'enabling the authorities to postpone decisions or avoid them altogether'. I warned:

> If the Commission fails to widen its brief, its work will be virtually irrelevant, and it will probably serve as a whitewash on the issue, whether the Commission intended it to or not.

Altogether, a most unsatisfactory situation. The Commission's report was due to be published at about the same time as this book. I would be happy to be shown to have misjudged the Commission, but I cannot see how, on the brief it devised for itself, its deliberations could change the status quo.

The European Factor

When the Prime Minister Mrs. Margaret Thatcher was confronted in the House of Commons in February 1982 by the leaders of the Labour and Liberal Parties, Michael Foot and David Steel, on the issue of lead-free petrol, it was noticeable that she did not choose to defend the 0.15 policy on the basis of the health evidence or indeed on any other of the arguments employed by her Health and Environmental Ministers; rather she chose the European factor.

The European factor, in a nutshell, is EEC Directive No. 78/611. This requires a maximum of 0.40 grams per litre and a minimum of 0.15 grams per litre for lead in petrol in Common Market countries. In other words, the EEC has ruled out in law any national regulations permitting lead-free petrol. This, as a matter of principle, should concern member countries. It surely does not make sense and it should not be the purpose of the EEC to actually ban measures that responsible public health authorities may wish to take in their country to protect their people from hazard.

What from the British point of view should, however, be of equal concern, is that Britain was the main opponent to the introduction of Directive 78/611, not because it wished to retain the flexibility to proceed to lead-free petrol, but because it wished to retain a minimum of 0.40 grams per litre!

Nigel Haigh, Programme Director of the European Environmental Policy Programme, wrote to *The Times* last year to describe the 'role the European Community has played in moving the UK faster than it wanted to'. He said:

> In 1973, when the EEC Commission proposed a directive making 0.4 grams of lead per litre the maximum permitted for sale in the Community, several European countries permitted up to 0.84 grams per litre and some had no limit at all.

The UK was already in the process of reducing its level from 0.84 when the Commission began its work, but both political parties here in the UK thought the Commission was moving too fast. The House of Commons, for example, resolved in 1976 'that this House accepts the principle of reducing the maximum lead content of petrol to 0.40 grams per litre . . . and, whilst recognising this will have an adverse effect on the United Kingdom's balance of payments, nevertheless calls on her Majesty's Government to achieve this aim by staged reductions.

The British Conservative Group voted against the directive in the European Parliament in 1975 and a Labour Minister, Denis Howell, was successful in delaying the reduction to 0.40 grams from 1977, the date originally proposed, to 1981.

Confronted in the House of Commons, Margaret Thatcher defended present policy in the European context with two points: first, that British cars, manufactured differently from European cars in order to run on lead-free petrol, would not sell on the European market, or would need to be adapted and that this would put the British car manufacturing industry at a disadvantage. Second, that Britain simply could not override the EEC Directive.

I wrote to the Prime Minister:

It is incorrect to say that British car manufacturers would be put at a disadvantage if they went alone. . . . How can they say that when one of the main problems is competition from the Japanese cars? The Japanese have been in no way hindered by the move to lead-free petrol; indeed their success has become an embarrassment to this country.

It is surely unacceptable to offer the EEC as an excuse for inaction when there is no evidence of this country campaigning in the EEC for a European approach. As you have named the EEC as one of the main obstacles to progress, surely the earliest possible instructions to Ministers to act would make sense.

At the time when you were fighting your totally just campaign for a better financial deal for Britain, you made it clear that Britain would be prepared to take unilateral steps to force the EEC to respond to the justice of your demands. Surely the health of our children is of equal importance, and you yourself have established a precedent for enforcing our opinion upon the EEC.

At the Liberal Party Assembly later in the year, delegates overwhelmingly defeated an amendment to a resolution calling for lead-free petrol. That amendment proposed negotiation with 'our European partners' rather than a unilateral decision. I pointed out that:

Tory Ministers will love it. It lets them off the hook. It means that the same lengthy debate that has taken place in Britain for over ten years will now need to take place in nine other countries – there will be the same lengthy deliberations, scientific sell-outs, industrial dishonesties, and all the time Britain's children will have to wait, despite the fact that we have convinced ourselves already that action should be taken. It's the way out for these Ministers. We must not let them off the hook. We must take the decision in this country about the health of our children and then set out to persuade to rest of Europe.

In addition, CLEAR drew attention to Article 36 of the Treaty of Rome. It states:

> The provisions of article 30–34 shall not preclude prohibitions or restrictions on imports, exports, or goods in transit justified on grounds of public morality, public policy or public security, *the protection of health and life of humans, animals, or plants*. . . .

Nevertheless, CLEAR decided it should launch a European initiative. Firstly, we engaged the support of Stanley Johnson, Conservative MEP who was Deputy Chairman of the European Parliament Environmental Committee. He tabled a resolution calling for moves to lead-free petrol, and this was then referred to the Environmental Committee, where a supporter of CLEAR, Ken Collins, Labour MEP from Scotland, was Johnson's Chairman. The Committee began an investigation into this problem.

In the meantime, I travelled twice to Brussels for meetings with the European Environmental Bureau and the Bureau of European Consumers' Unions (the EEB and BEUC). These two organisations coordinate in Brussels the EEC campaigning activities of environmental and consumer organisations throughout Europe. There had always been some rivalry between them and they had never campaigned jointly before, but they were persuaded to join together in a major European campaign to be launched in October 1982.

A first-class report was prepared by the two organisations. It argued that Europe had always been slow to follow the movement towards lead-free petrol:

> . . . It would not enhance the diminishing popularity of the EEC if it were to appear as an obstacle to progress not only for its own citizens, but also to other European neighbouring countries.

The European campaign was launched in Brussels on October 28 at a press conference staged by the EEB and BEUC with myself present. On the same day a press conference was held in most of the other major European capitals, including London where the

Consumer's Association and the National Consumer Council, until then subdued on the issue, finally committed themselves to the cause.

A representative of the National Consumer Council stated:

> We believe that the question that now needs to be asked is not whether we should get lead out of petrol, but how.

He argued that Britain should seek to change European legislation.

> We are never likely to make the oil and motor industries willing partners in this change-over if we try to take action only on a national basis.

The launch of this campaign represent a considerable achievement for CLEAR and a source of additional embarrassment for British Ministers.

Into 1983 . . . The State of Play

As 1982 came to an end CLEAR achieved one major success with the disclosure by the can manufacturing industry that it was eliminating all lead solder from its product as a result of public concern over lead pollution. The BBC TV programme 'Newsnight' pointed out to Giles Shaw during a special film on lead in petrol that he had become totally isolated on the issue. Shaw remained as stubborn as ever. Associated Octel wrote to *The Guardian* to say that blood-lead levels in Britain were low and the problem of lead pollution exaggerated. As for CLEAR – it began to lay plans for what would probably be an election year campaign in 1983. . . .

7.
The guilty ones

Broadly speaking, I try to be a believer in the cock-up theory of political life, rather than the conspiracy theory. In other words, I tend to assume that bad decisions are caused by error, mischance, misunderstanding, or stupidity, rather than corruption, self-service or malice.

This controversy has had its share of accusation and suspicion, but there is little need to be imaginative. There were five contributors to the May 1981 decision – the petroleum industry, the car manufacturers, Associated Octel, the scientists, and the politicians (together with their civil servants) – and, on the evidence, all deserve censure.

The scientific community is at fault because it participated in the creation of an unbalanced working party in the Lawther Committee and this not surprisingly produced an unbalanced report. While a number of the working party were known to hold firm views supportive of the use of lead in petrol, all those known to have firm views on the other side were excluded. The scientific community has demonstrably put a far greater burden of proof on those who claimed a health hazard, than on the industries to establish safety. It has demanded a far greater weight of evidence of health hazard than prudence would demand. It has tended to be over-influenced by economic considerations that were none of its business. Its failure to spot the hazard for so many decades and its reluctance to accept the accumulating evidence has been as unimpressive as the undisguised predilection of some of its number to challenge and dispute and undermine each study as it has appeared.

It is hardly a coincidence that the industries with a vested interest in the decision have been united in refusing to accept the evidence of a health hazard. They have spent considerable sums of money fighting lead-free petrol. With these industries, profit has come before people. They do not accept any responsibility to the citizen or the community. They repeatedly state that the debate on the health hazard is not within their province, yet no-one should have the right to make and manufacture a product without proving that it is safe, nor to stubbornly pursue a practice that is said to be dangerous and wash their hands completely of the repercussions by stating that they are not qualified to judge the issue.

The politicians over-ruled in May 1981 the advice of the Ministries most concerned with environmental protection, health and education. They did this after lengthy deliberations with the car manufacturing and petroleum industries and took a short-term decision based on economics and the interests of the multi-nationals. Having taken that decision, they closed their minds to all the additional evidence that has emerged and to the growing concern of the public, and decided to obstinately carry on, calculating that they could get away with it.

The failure to get lead out of petrol does, therefore, extend beyond the 'cock-up' explanation. In the case of the industries, they have been cynical and selfish. In the case of at least some scientists, they simply don't wish to admit they have been at fault. In the case of the politicians and public health authorities, they are open to the serious charge that they are actually fighting a campaign to protect lead in petrol with the same determination that the majority of their fellow citizens are fighting to protect public health.

Let's examine the role and behaviour of each of these in detail.

The Petroleum Industry

The petroleum industry in Britain has endeavoured since the launch of the CLEAR campaign to paint itself whiter than white. Its claims can be summed up as follows:

(1)   It is not qualified to comment on the health evidence, but will respond positively to whatever legislation is introduced. It is, therefore, neutral on the health issue.

(2)   It actually offered lead-free petrol to Whitehall in 1980–81 and was rejected, and cannot be blamed for the decision to reduce to only 0.15 grams per litre.

In every respect, this position is duplicitous. During the Albery case, the petroleum industry produced witnesses to directly challenge the evidence of health risk. Furthermore, the petroleum industry owns Associated Octel, who have been remorseless in their efforts to claim there is no health risk whatsoever, and it has not attempted to modify Octel's activities; on the contrary, Octel has steadily increased its defensive activities (as I will demonstrate later) and the petroleum industry has been happy for Octel to do its dirty work.

On the question of whether it wants lead-free petrol, the petroleum industry has played a double game. It has never publicly called for lead-free petrol, never assisted or supported the anti-lead movement in any way, and in fact, has conducted a public relations campaign calculated to present itself in the best possible light whilst producing as many obstacles to lead-free petrol as it possibly could. Unlike some petroleum companies in the United States, not one petroleum company in Britain has produced lead-free petrol before being forced to do so by legislation. It is indeed the case that the petroleum industry offered lead-free petrol to Whitehall in 1980–81. But this was done behind closed doors, never voluntarily made public, and the offer was one the petroleum industry was confident the car manufacturers would oppose, because the offer was low octane petrol whereas the car manufacturing industry was producing vehicles made to run on high octane petrol. In other words, the petroleum industry 'set up' the car manufacturing industry as the obstacle to progress.

Furthermore, the petroleum industry did not in fact *press* for lead-free petrol in 1981. They argued that *if* it was planned to move to lead-free petrol eventually, they would rather do it immediately in order to avoid the intermediate costs of transition to 0.15. In this way they were able to obtain an informal understanding that if they shouldered the costs of a reduction to 0.15, the Government would not fix a further date for a move to lead-free petrol.

The whole history of this issue all over the world has been marked by the fight of the petroleum companies against a ban on lead. As we saw in Chapter One, the US petroleum companies (many of them the same companies operating in Britain) did all in their power to prevent regulation or to have regulations overthrown. Clarence Ditlow, chief of Ralph Nader's auto safety campaign in the United States, says 'the oil companies fought lead regulation tooth and nail over the years'. Their economic forecasts in several countries have proved wildly exaggerated. The Australian Institute of Petroleum spent about $250,000 on a campaign to stop the decision to move to unleaded petrol. A report by the Vehicle Emissions and Noise Standards Committee said that early in 1980 the oil companies put the transition cost at $400 million. This was later reduced to $300 million. Five months later it was reduced to $195 million. Still the Committee found scope for significant reductions in the figure. It concluded that the oil industry estimates were exaggerated more than 10 times!

In West Germany, the petroleum industry estimated the cost of reducing the lead levels in petrol to 0.15 grams per litre at DM1,000 million for modifications in refineries; all 25 refineries were modified and the actual cost was well under DM300 million – less than a third of the figure the industry had projected. The German petroleum industry warned of increased prices but the German delegation to the UN Environmental Programme seminar on the petroleum industry in 1977 stated that 'there was no basis to attributing any real price increases to the reduction of lead' and that 'as a whole it was found that the fears of negative consequences in various respects which had been canvassed before the decree was implemented proved to be greatly exaggerated'.

Prior to the final decision on the launching of CLEAR, on November 9, 1981, I wrote letters to 10 leading British oil companies on behalf of 'a number of individuals concerned about the growing body of evidence of a serious health hazard arising from the use of lead in petrol', and I sought further clarification of the individual companies' position and the answers to a number of technical questions. I also requested that the companies meet a deputation to discuss the issue further.

Not one of the ten companies would answer the questions, or meet the deputation.

Every one of the ten companies wrote an almost identical letter saying that we would be answered by the UK Petroleum Industry Association. (It took *ten weeks* for the reply from the Association to arrive, and when it did, it consisted of a few trite phrases that could have been drafted overnight.)

What was astonishing was the communication that had quickly taken place between the companies, as reflected in the letters received:

For instance, Conoco Limited wrote: 'This is a matter that the UK Petroleum Industry Association keeps under review *and I understand that they will be responding to you in due course*'.

BP wrote: '*I understand you have addressed similar letters to other oil companies* . . . the Petroleum Industry Association will be replying very shortly with a full response to the points you raise.'

Shell wrote: 'The points you raise are being dealt with by the Petroleum Industry Association UKPIA; it is probably better that they respond and *I understand that they intend to do so*'.

A number of points need to be made about this:

First, while there probably is an overall industry point of view on this issue and there is no reason why the PIA should not state it, it is inconceivable that each company does not have its own view on any question affecting it, let alone a question of such importance. Furthermore no individual company can evade its own responsibility on issues of public health and safety.

Second, the similarity of the replies received from all 10 companies together with open admission of knowledge by each company that it knew other companies had been approached and that the Association was responding on their behalf, shows the defensive mechanism which exists on the issue. It is disturbing that huge and wealthy companies, confronted with a simple set of questions from a private individual writing on behalf of other individuals, should mobilise such a well coordinated response. Their letters made clear that the telephones buzzed between them and their Association. If they do this in reply to one letter, from one person, it is worth asking what defence mechanism they set up when they feel themselves under *real* pressure – for instance when they are faced with enquiries from Whitehall?

Third, the refusal of all 10 companies to even consider meeting a deputation on a matter of such deep public concern reflects their priorities and the little time they are prepared to set aside to communicate with people other than those who – we must assume – can contribute to their profits.

Fourth, the only possible assumption that can be made is that all of the companies were concerned that they should not inadvertently make a concession on the economics and technical details that would contradict the centrally-organised line of the public-relations-orientated UK Petroleum Industry Association.

Further evidence of their attitude is their position on evidence to the Royal Commission on Environmental Pollution. When in 1982 CLEAR submitted its evidence, we sent that evidence to every commercial, voluntary, and Governmental organisation listed as having been invited to testify. We had sufficient confidence in our evidence to do that. In return, we invited each of these organisations to send a copy of their evidence to CLEAR. Most did so, including Ministries. The only refusals we received were from the lead industry and the petroleum industry. As I pointed out at the time, this was not a matter of national security but a matter of public health. The behaviour of the petroleum industry in refusing to share its evidence was extraordinary. It reflects both its arrogance, and its lack of confidence that its evidence would withstand the public spotlight.

The front man for the petroleum industry is Douglas Harvey, Director of the UK Petroleum Industry Association. In an article in *Consumer Affairs* in July/August 1982 he demonstrated the way the petroleum industry likes to play its hand on the question of public health; 'The health evidence which the campaign quotes is at best inconclusive', he said. Harvey had attended the CLEAR symposium and heard the evidence and heard the Rutter summing-up. Yet he still was demanding conclusive evidence and his reference to 'at best inconclusive' was calculated to imply that it was probably worse. This is typical of the way Harvey and the petroleum industry always refer to the health evidence.

In any case, the petroleum industry's position that it is not for them to reach conclusions about the health risk is unacceptable. If one follows that argument to its logical conclusion then anyone is entitled to perform any act, no matter how dangerous, until such time as the authorities order it otherwise. Not only has the petroleum industry not been neutral on the health question, but nor should it be. It has a responsibility to be fully involved, to explore the health risk it creates, and to enter the debate on it. If it does not, it is in effect saying that its concern is the making of money, and responsibility for the health of human beings belongs elsewhere. No individual, no company, can properly assume such a position. The petroleum industry has an enormous vested interest – the saving of money and the making of profit. The petroleum industry's position is clear: it could produce low octane petrol quickly and cheaply, and when in 1980–1 it was confronted with the probability of a reduction to 0.15 grams per litre with the possibility of a further reduction later to lead-free petrol, it decided to abandon the car manufacturing industry, with whom to that point it had shared a common policy of furthering a monopoly of high-compression engines.

It knew that its offer of low octane lead-free petrol achieved the best of all possible worlds. First, if this was decided upon, it would avoid the transition costs to 0.15 grams per litre. If, on the other hand, it was decided not to proceed to lead-free petrol, the petroleum industry could claim that its hands were clean, and that the car manufacturing industry was the villain of the piece. Thus Harvey was able to say in an article for *Consumer Affairs*:

> Far from conspiring to retain lead in petrol, the oil industry recommended last year that, if it were decided that lead levels should be further reduced, the best way of doing so was to introduce unleaded petrol (2-star) as soon as possible. The car population could then progressively switch to this as new cars, designed to run on 2-star, replaced existing cars.

Typical of the attitude of the petroleum industry to the public is the secrecy that surrounded their offer of lead-free petrol. When Tom King announced in the House of Commons in May 1981 the decision to reduce to 0.15 grams per litre, few, if any, Members of Parliament who questioned him knew that the petroleum industry had offered lead-free petrol. When CLEAR was launched in January 1982 this was still unknown, but one of the benefits of the CLEAR campaign is that both the petroleum and car manufacturing industries have been embarrassed into disclosures that they would have preferred not to make. In the case of BP, for instance, they became sufficiently embarrassed by the criticisms of petroleum companies to issue an internal memorandum to staff. This was leaked to CLEAR. And it contained the confession:

> The oil industry recommended last year that, if it was decided that lead levels should be further reduced, the best way of doing so was to introduce unleaded petrol (2-star) as soon as possible. The car population could then progressively switch to this as new cars (designed to run on 2-star) replaced existing cars.

(Notice that this is exactly the same wording that Harvey was to later use in the *Consumer Affairs* article quoted earlier, yet more evidence of the care all these massive companies take to correlate what they say. Also in the document BP said 'Lead-free petrol at 2-star octane levels would cost only a few pence more to produce than the equivalent leaded grade'. Harvey in his later article in *Consumer Affairs* said 'Lead-free petrol at 2-star octane levels would cost only a few pence more to produce than the equivalent leaded grade'. The same words.)

BP also said:

> The oil industry could produce this type of petrol after only a short delay. Further, most current 2-star engines have been designed to run on it, although the car industry would need time to shift production from the 4-star designs that predominate at the moment. 4-star leaded petrol would also have to be retained for some years for the present generation of cars that can run on it alone.

In other words, BP was really letting the cat out of the bag, at the same time confirming that CLEAR's objectives of a phasing-out of lead in petrol were perfectly possible.

I subsequently wrote to Harvey and asked him to clarify whether or not the petroleum industry still wanted to move directly to lead-free petrol. But already money was talking. Some of it had been invested in the move to 0.15 grams per litre so Harvey was no longer able to take such a firm line as a definite recommendation to move directly to lead-free:

> We confirm that we indicated to HMG, prior to their May 1981 decision, that if the choice lay between introduction of unleaded low octane petrol and a reduction in lead additives from 0.4 grams per litre to 0.15 grams per litre in all petrol, then we would prefer the former. . . . However, following Government adoption of the 0.15 grams per litre maintained octane route, the industry is now deeply involved in refinery adaptations necessary to implementation of that decision.

He also claimed:

In general engineering-processing-project planning to implement the move to 0.15 grams per litre is well advanced, with substantial related financial commitments.

Unfortunately, the petroleum companies alone control the information on costs and technical matters, and it is almost impossible to cross-check what they say. When it was announced that we were to proceed to 0.15 grams per litre by the end of 1985, Texaco announced that it did not have capability to produce 0.15 grams per litre at current octane levels in the volume required for its sales in the UK and would need to spend more on processing equipment. 'In view of the new processing facilities required it is unlikely that Texaco would be prepared to market the reduced lead petrol in advance of the mandated date which was in fact designed to permit adequate time for the oil industry to adjust production to the new lead level.' Thus, it was clear, that Texaco intended to wait until 1985 before reducing to 0.15 grams per litre.

In contrast to this, Martin Stevens, MP, after conversations with Tom King, wrote to Bob Stephens to say, 'The Minister is confident that they can reach 0.15 grams per litre well before the December 1985 deadline'.

In many ways I find the behaviour of the petroleum industry the most reprehensible of the three industries involved. Whilst the car manufacturers are guilty of putting their narrow financial concerns before the health of children, they are at least open about it. Octel are more than open – they are flagrant. The petroleum industry, however, has tried to play it both ways, on the one hand apparently eager and willing to do what is required, and on the other, relying on the car manufacturers to make the substantial case for the status quo and Associated Octel to do the dirty work of denying the health risk.

They arrogantly seek to exclude the public from the debate. They go to absurd lengths to cover their tracks and ensure they are all telling the same story. The fact is that they own the company that manufactures the poisonous product, they add that product to their own, and then they claim that the health issue is not their responsibility. As I said when CLEAR was launched, 'Be in no doubt what we are saying about the petroleum companies: we are saying that they are adding to their product a known neurotoxin and that they know that it is widely dispersed into the air from exhaust pipes, and that there is increasing evidence that it puts the nation's children at risk. We are saying they are gambling with arrogance and cynicism that the ill-effects are minimal, knowing that if they are eventually proven – as we believe they already are – to be wrong, there will be no dead bodies to point to, few children could prove conclusively in a court of law that their problems were caused only by lead, and that because their guilt is shared with other industries and with civil servants and politicians who have delayed action, the change to lead-free petrol, when it comes, will be carried out with the minimum of blame being attached to them.'

Associated Octel

The Associated Octel Company Limited at Ellesmere Port is the sole British manufacturer of lead additives to petrol. Over 80% of its product is exported and for its contribution to extending this hazard to children across the globe it has won two Queen's awards for export achievement. The company is proud of what it does. Under pressure from CLEAR, the company in September 1982 spent at least £100,000 on full-page advertising in *The Times*, *Guardian*, *Daily Telegraph*, *Observer*, and *Sunday Times*, describing its 'achievements' under the headline 'The Health and Wealth of the Nation'.

Octel is the creature of the oil companies. It is wholly owned by a consortium of BP, Shell, Mobil, Chevron, and Texaco, in the form of the Anglo-Saxon Petroleum Company (address: Shell Centre, London), Dorchester Oil Trading Company Limited (address: BP House, London), Chevron Oceanic Inc (New York), Texaco International Trading Inc (New York), Mobil Holdings Limited (London) and Shell UK Limited (London). Its directors, at least until recently, included such as G. S. Simpson (other director-ships – Shell Holdings UK Limited, Shell UK Limited, Shell Mex and BP Pension and Provident Fund Limited, Irish Shell Limited, Irish Shell Trust Limited), I. R. Walker (UK Petroleum Industry Association Limited, BP Oil Limited, BP Oil Grangemouth Refinery Limited, BP Oil Kent Refinery Limited, BP Oil Northern Ireland Refinery Limited, Scottish Oils Limited, BP Detergents Limited) and J. W. Patterson (Shell Research Limited, Shell Gases Limited, Shell UK Exploration and Production Limited, Shell Refining and Marketing Limited). Walker's directorship of the United Kingdom Petroleum Industry Association Limited is particularly noteworthy for it raises a further question over the so-called neutrality of that organisation on the lead-in-petrol issue. Octel owns three other companies – Octel Societe Anonyme in France, A. K. Chemie GmbH in Germany, and A. K. Chemie GmbH & Co. KG in

Germany. In 1979 it declared a profit before taxation of £6,822,000 and total retained profits of £1,817,000. The decision to reduce to 0.15 grams per litre by 1985 was expected to reduce its manufacturing capacity by 11½%.

In 1975 909 drums of tetraethyl and tetramethyl lead from Associated Octel were deposited on the floor of the Mediterranean when their carrier ship sank. Jacques Cousteau described it as 'a poisonous bomb, full of death, momentarily asleep'. *The Sunday Times* reported it as 'a poison timebomb'. Associated Octel's technical manager in Rome was quoted as saying 'We have absolutely no interest in raising this ship. We don't own anything. We don't want anything.' For a time there was an attempt to cover up the whole affair. *The Sunday Times* obtained a three-page memorandum written by an Associated Octel executive in April 1975. It was quoted as saying: 'After a long period in the sea, corrosion will result in leaks and anti-knock compound will escape into the sea. It is not possible to predict with any accuracy the time required for all 900 drums to empty but it could be as long as ten years.' The Italian authorities were thinking of raising the cargo but Octel's memorandum stated: 'We have advised the authorities that the best course of action is to leave the ship and cargo where they are. Salvage of any or all of the cargo from such deep water will be difficult and possibly dangerous.' *The Sunday Times* stated that 'The poison drums present a terrifying Catch-22 situation. They may be too dangerous to be salvaged and at the same time too dangerous to be left where they are.'

Two years later Octel's deadly poison still lay at the bottom of the Mediterranean, threatening, should the drums begin to leak, what *The Observer* reported scientists and marine biologists describing as 'an ecological catastrophe to human and marine life in the Mediterranean'. Fish wholesalers in the area found they could no longer sell their products. 'Luckily our fish doesn't carry any labels' said a fish merchant. A leading University Professor in Rome stated: 'You would want your head examined if you go swimming in the sea near there'. There was a deluge of cancellations from local hotels. While the Italian authorities were left with the headaches and the costs of the problems, Associated Octel simply washed their hands of the whole affair. The Italians eventually spent millions salvaging the drums.

Unlike the petroleum industry, but on its behalf, Associated Octel has entered the debate on the health hazard with vigour, producing propaganda calculated to contradict the evidence of risk and spending a considerable sum of money on scientists who it would present as 'leading experts' on lead and health.

As far back as 1976 it was resisting any reduction. For instance, on March 3, 1976, the following notice appeared on works notice boards in Associated Octel's factories:

Notice – Lead in Petrol
On Thursday, 4th March, 1976, the House of Commons will have before it a motion concerning the EEC proposals for the phased reduction of lead in petrol.
The company's activities over a wide field covering Government Departments, research establishments, contacts with MPs (both UK and EEC) etc, *to resist these proposals* have been made known, from time to time, through our established consultative channels. These will be reiterated by Departmental and Works Managers, as far as possible, to individual employees during the next day or so.
Those employees who have a particular interest in the present situation and, for various reasons, have been unable to obtain the current information, are asked to contact their supervisor. Arrangements will be made for this information to be made available.

F. Smith

Particularly noteworthy is the reference to 'the company's activities' covering 'research establishments' to 'resist these proposals'. This makes nonsense of Octel's claim to undertake objective research and makes clear that their so-called research activities are in fact designed for one reason only – to resist any proposal for the reduction of lead in petrol.

As it became clear in 1982 that the campaign by CLEAR was making substantial inroads into its credibility, Octel moved its 'heavy', Peter Dartnell, into control of 'public affairs' and set aside a considerable sum of money for advertising, leaflets, factory visits, massive entertaining of MPs, local councillors, and anyone else who would listen, in a determined effort to protect its profits.

One of its leading defenders was for years its 'chief medical officer', Dr. P. S. I. Barry, whose signature frequently appeared under letters or articles designed to allay fears about the health risk involved. Barry qualified as a medical practitioner and joined Octel virtually immediately. He worked for the company for 30 years. In 1982 Octel was embarrassed in *The Lancet* when Barry attempted to distort the work of a distinguished overseas scientist and was exposed by that scientist.

Dr. Robin Russell Jones had written to *The Lancet* and stated that the consensus of medical opinion on the lead in petrol issue had shifted significantly. He specifically referred to the position of Dr. Gerhard Winneke, the respected German scientist.

On July 10 Barry wrote to *The Lancet* to say . . .

the truth is not as he would have it. . . . . One speaker, Dr. G. Winneke, failed to support the CLEAR position. Winneke rescinded the preliminary results of his earlier studies in the light of his own new evidence, and showed that socio-hereditary factors were principally responsible for the adverse effects observed in children, and not lead. Russell Jones does not mention this embarrassing change in evidence. Furthermore, Winneke stated that he did not believe the animal experiments to be relevant to human lead exposure; Russell Jones implies that Winneke said the opposite.

On September 4, Winneke wrote to *The Lancet*:

Barry claims that I 'rescinded the preliminary results of my earlier studies in the light of my new evidence that socio-hereditary factors were principally responsible for the adverse effects observed in children and not lead' and that I do not believe the animal experiments to be relevant to human lead exposure.

The truth is not as Barry would have it, as my paper and the original reports from our laboratory show. The important aspect of our new findings in lead-exposed children is that, apart from the well known strong influence of socio-hereditary background, environmental lead does seem to exert an additional detrimental effect on various neuro-psychological functions, most pronounced for visual-motor integration, behaviour ratings, and reaction performance, though not for intelligence after correcting for confounding. Our latest findings of significant visual-motor deficit confirm preliminary results from a pilot study. I pointed out at the CLEAR symposium that our animal data could not be extrapolated quantitively to man but that we regard them as highly relevant for cause-effect considerations as well as for clarifying the spectrum of neurobehavioural effects.

This state of affairs clearly does not correspond to the impression left by Barry's letter.

Octel produced a document from Barry commenting in detail on the Bryce-Smith/Stephens report, 'Lead or Health'. In the course of a nit-picking report questioning every bit of evidence except that supportive of Octel, he complained of 'unscientific' content or 'derogatory' comments in the Bryce-Smith/Stephens document and yet was exceptionally abusive himself.

A typical Barry comment in this document about Bryce-Smith and Stephens was: 'The impression given is one of self-opinionated arrogance, lacking entirely in objectivity or in any depth of knowledge which might have given some support, at least, to the authors' opinions.' He referred to various aspects of the Patterson work as 'The Patterson mythology' Other references to Bryce-Smith and

Stephens: 'This is a further example of the exaggeration devoid of practicalities that pervades the whole of the report. By the spurious use of some conjectural mathematics, the authors arrive at a supposed lead intake in children. . . .' 'Much of the discussion in this section is based on false information and is speculative in nature.'

While Barry was attempting to cover-up the health risks, Octel's 'heavy' in the political arena, Peter Dartnell, published his advertising 'The Health and Wealth of the Nation'. In a letter to *The Observer* I listed just three of its distortions:

1   It stated that assertions of 'a connection between airborne lead and health – and children's health in particular – are unsubstantiated medically or scientifically'. In fact a series of scientific studies recently convinced the US Environmental Protection Agency to step up still further their controls on lead in petrol. These studies would convince anyone who has no financial vested interest in the issue.

2   'Without lead, we would only be able to manufacture 2-star petrol'. This is nonsense. In the United States you can buy either regular or super unleaded fuel i.e. low octane and high octane.

3   'Present exhaust emissions from petrol produce only about 10% of body lead content.' Octel are the only people in the country left defending this figure. Even Ministers say it is 20% and the scientific evidence suggests between 30 and 60%.

A classic Dartnell quote can be found in the *Radio Times*: 'Lead in petrol in no way enhances the amount of lead in our blood'. The Government (under-estimate) figure is 20% and even Octel admits to 10%!

In March 1981 in the magazine, *Chemistry in Britain* Dr. D. Turner, who travels the country presenting Octel's defence at seminars, stated:

There is no evidence, however, that airborne lead from petrol has been the cause of ill health in any group of the general population, even in towns with heavy traffic. . . . It is much easier to produce evidence that suggests that there may be a risk than to produce positive proof that there is not – no-one has proved that ghosts do not exist!.

After the publication of the CLEAR handbook and the launch of CLEAR, Octel produced a leaflet entitled 'Lead in Petrol. . . . The Issues and the Facts' to answer what it described as 'a clamorous, self-appointed lobby' whose efforts it described as 'misguided and certainly uninformed'.

It made enormous play of the Lawther report, identifying Lawther, Barltrop and Clayton as particular experts, and then on the question of sources of exposure, it says of the CLEAR handbook:

On pages 10 and 11 great emphasis is given to the statement that 90% of airborne lead comes from car exhausts. Yet nowhere is it stated that lead from car exhausts makes up only 8% of the total lead burden, a fact which puts the whole issue back into perspective.

This figure of 8% of course has no more scientific basis than Octel's own more recent figure of 10%.

What is noticeable is that there is not one reference in the Octel pamphlets to the Needleman research, or the Yule and Lansdown study in Greenwich, or the Winneke study in Germany, or the Otto study, or indeed any of the other studies that have convinced the majority of responsible scientists that there is indeed a health case to answer. If Octel felt even minimal responsibility for public health it should at least answer these studies in its own material.

Despite its huge expenditure, Octel were, by the autumn of 1982, clearly losing their battle to cover up the health risk. For instance, despite the fact that full-page ads appeared in *The Guardian, The Times,* and *The Daily Telegraph* opposite reports of the Liberal Party Assembly in order that delegates could read them prior to the Assembly debate on lead in petrol, the Assembly voted almost unanimously for the earliest possible ban. So now the company began to change its tune, insisting that motorists should spend a considerable sum of money to buy an Octel-devised filter to protect children from a health risk that Octel still claimed did not exist.

As 1982 progressed Octel spent a fortune in new leaflets, in wining and dining MPs at Lockett's restaurant in London, and entertaining European MPs in Strasburg, and in advertising and promoting the filter. They claimed it had been 'independently' assessed by Government scientists at Harwell. CLEAR advised rejection of the filter on the following grounds:

1   *Rejected by all other countries*
The United States, Japan, and now Australia, three countries phasing out lead in petrol, all seriously considered filters as an alternative to lead-free petrol and rejected them. Germany also considered and rejected filters as did the UK authorities at the time the decision was taken to reduce lead in petrol to 0.15 grams per litre. All have rejected filters for the same reasons:

● they are expensive
● they are only partly efficient – they do not catch all the lead, and furthermore, they only achieve their maximum potential under some driving conditions
● their efficiency deteriorates with age and it is impossible to enforce maintenance
● there is a disposal problem

Furthermore, for those countries wishing to control emissions of other pollutants, leaded petrol prevents the use of catalytic converters.

2   They are inefficient

Octel's publication entitled 'Vehicle Exhaust Gas Filters' states that the filters will 'reduce lead emissions by up to 60% averaged over all driving conditions'. This is clearly not good enough. As the Environmental Protection Agency in the USA has concluded, lead in petrol contributes 46% of lead intake and up to two-thirds of the lead intake for some urban children; any proposal only seeking to reduce lead emissions in part does not represent an adequate response to the medical and scientific data. Even greater efficiencies have been recently claimed by Associated Octel but these claims are not borne out by closer inspection of the published document (Atomic Energy Research Establishment, Harwell, document G2474). Both the filters tested were relatively new and in one case had been driven less than 10,000 miles. No-one denies that filters may be fairly effective initially. The point at issue is whether their efficiency deteriorates with use. It is therefore significant that lead emissions from older filters (17,000 miles) were erratic and under one set of driving conditions did not differ significantly from untrapped vehicles. Furthermore, the overall efficiency of the 17,000 mile filter was only 50%. Far from demonstrating the efficiency of filters, the Harwell data confirms that the filters become inefficient with age and that this deterioration occurs fairly early on in the filter's life.

It is significant that an Associated Octel employee has circulated a document stating, 'I am of the opinion that this filter, while it reduces the lead content in the exhaust gas, doesn't solve the real pollution problem.'

3   How independent was the Harwell report?

Although the Harwell document was presented by Octel as independently assessing its filter, certain procedures were carried out which seriously undermine the independence of the report. First, the Harwell team had no independent verification that the filters had in fact been driven for the mileages stated. Second, half the measurements in these experiments were carried out by staff at Associated Octel's laboratory. The fact that the company has a huge vested interest in the results of this research does not in itself mean the results were suspect; what it does mean, however, is that the Harwell report does not represent a totally independent assessment of the filter. Furthermore, there are anomalies in the presentation of the data which have not been adequately explained. First, the Harwell research team does not even mention, let alone discuss, the deterioration of the efficiency of the filters with age. Instead, it pools all the results and arrives at an overall efficiency for the filter without pointing out that the older filter is considerably less efficient than the new filter. Even more serious is that the older filter is tested under three separate driving conditions but four sets of results are included in the final analysis, two of which were obtained under the least strenuous driving conditions. In other words, the apparent efficiency of the filter has been artificially improved by pooling all the results and then giving unequal weight to the more favourable results.

4   Organo-lead emissions

Car exhausts emit two types of lead. The major part is inorganic lead which is emitted as lead particulates and these are the particulates supposed to be trapped by the lead filter. However, uncombusted tetraethyl lead (organic lead) is emitted as a vapour and in urban driving conditions may account for as much as 10% of atmospheric lead. Organo-lead emissions are approximately ten times as dangerous as inorganic lead and there is no evidence that the filter has a significant effect on their concentration in urban air.

5   No help to the motorist

If we move to lead-free petrol, the motorist will obtain positive advantages in lower maintenance costs and less engine wear. These benefits would be lost by the use of the filter.

6   No answer to international markets

British car manufacturers already supply cars for the United States and Japan to run on lead-free petrol and will shortly have to do so for Australia. There is already a powerful initiative in the EEC for a move throughout Europe to lead-free petrol. It is a patent absurdity for British industry to be grasping at a half-way solution when there is an outstanding opportunity to anticipate international demand for a permanent solution to a major environmental problem.

7   Who will benefit?

Even if the filter will reduce airborne lead emissions, and no doubt it will to some extent, who will benefit most? Surely the answer is Associated Octel.

No-one will benefit from the continuation of the build-up of lead in the environment.

No-one will benefit from the extra financial cost of the filters.

No-one will benefit from the engine damage that lead continues to cause.

No-one will ultimately benefit from a half-measure in response to the evidence of health damage.

No-one will benefit from introducing a filter that quickly becomes outdated as other countries accept, as one day they must do, the nature of the health hazard and the need for comprehensive action.

As 1982 proceeded Octel continued its desperate search for any scrap of scientific material, no matter how obscure the source, to strengthen its claims that its product was safe, and that there was no cause for concern. No doubt it will continue to do so. But does it believe its own story? Does the Board of Octel, and do its senior executives, suffer from the understandable human tendency to believe what they want to believe? Are they wrong, but innocently so? This would be the charitable view, but the one-sided nature of their propaganda, the selectivity adopted in the scientific material they quote, and the transparent distortion of the facts is systematic and sustained. When one day it is widely understood and accepted that the use of lead in petrol has done considerable damage to generations of children, it is hard to see how they could have any defence.

The Car Manufacturers

At the same time as I wrote to the petroleum industry in 1981, I also wrote with a list of questions to car manufacturers. One, Talbot, attempted the same approach as the oil companies – 'I feel your questionnaire can be better handled on an industry-wide basis. Accordingly perhaps I could suggest you contact the Society of Motor Manufacturers and Traders'. Reliant wrote that 'a letter without formal heading from a private individual, rather than an association . . . does not necessarily warrant a great deal of time or attention'.

To begin at the top end of the market, Rolls Royce indicated that 42% of its vehicles were already manufactured to run on lead-free petrol because they were 'sold in markets where lead-free petrol is used'. Cars sold in the USA which run on lead-free fuel were designed with an octane rating of 91. 'We reduce the compression ratio and modify the ignition timing and other engine tuning parameters to suit the lower octane rating.'

Still at the top end of the market, Lotus wrote to say that their cars did not need leaded petrol. 'As our engines do not need lead we have no position on when a move to lead-free fuel is made.'

Moving to the market more appropriate for the bulk of motorists, Sam Toy of Ford wrote:

Whilst acknowledging the purpose of lead in petrol, Ford has for some time been concerned about its possible ill effects – even though there has been and still is a considerable controversy about what those effects might be. Since August 1976 we have engineered and manufactured vehicles to run on 0.15 grams per litre. Should the Government decide to mandate lead-free fuel for motor vehicles then all we ask is for sufficient time to be allowed for us to obtain the money and other resources to make the changes.

On how long it would take to re-design, re-test and re-tool Ford's engines and vehicles to run on lead-free petrol, Toy said it could 'not be practically undertaken in less than five years'.

Vauxhall replied that . . .

all the cars we are currently making and selling have been engineered to meet the lead additive limit of 0.15 grams per litre. . . . The technology is also available for the production of engines that will operate on lead-free petrol. . . . In summary, the technology for reducing or eliminating lead exists, but the on-cost in terms of vehicles and fuel would have marked economic implications.

British Leyland replied:

I am sure you appreciate that British Leyland is not qualified to express or assess views on the relationships between lead levels in petrol and public health. We have been, and must continue to be, guided by Government legislation and we believe it is the Government's responsibility to consider all the evidence and determine whether further action is required to limit lead levels in petrol; we will cooperate willingly should such a decision be taken, provided that adequate notice of implementation is given.

British Leyland emphasised that 'there are no great technical problems in producing new car engines to run on lead-free petrol, and provided the octane number of the fuel is maintained, the cost of doing so is comparatively modest'. They emphasised however that the octane number was critical. If a lower octane route was taken 'most current engines would have to be redeveloped, production modifications introduced, and the engines and models concerned resubmitted through the whole cycle of mandatory Government test procedures'. 'A period of notice, of about five years, would be needed for any move to lead-free petrol.'

British Leyland confirmed that they were manufacturing cars to run on lead-free petrol for both the USA and Japan.

The first point to be made about these replies was that the car manufacturers had at least responded more openly than the petroleum industry. British Leyland, however, had taken the same position as the oil industry, namely that the public health question was not for the industry to consider. I can only repeat my view that no industry is entitled to reject all responsibility for the effects of its actions.

Most notable, however, was that whereas the petroleum industry had emphasised in all its pronouncements that the only possible option was low octane fuel, the car manufacturers suggested that there would be no problems for them if the high octane route was taken, thus making it clear that both industries have to some extent sheltered behind the known objection of the other to one of the two alternative routes. As the strength of the car manufacturers' feelings about a loss of high octane petrol emerged, it became even clearer why the petroleum industry felt safe to offer low octane petrol to Ministers in 1980–81; they knew only too well the strength of the opposite case being put by the car manufacturers.

In the middle of 1982 a supporter of CLEAR, Mrs. Ruth Savery, wrote to a number of car manufacturers 'as a mother of young children living in an area of high traffic density' to enquire about the potential of the companies to produce cars to run on lead-free petrol. The replies were fascinating. British Leyland replied with their standard line about not being 'qualified to express any view on the relationship between lead levels in petrol and public health' but said

> As to whether BL should independently introduce cars that run on lead-free petrol, the answer is that some of our engines will already basically function satisfactorily on unleaded fuel, although there are other engines which require production modifications. However, there is little point at present in undertaking this work since lead-free fuel is not available in the UK.

(Now we had a situation where the petroleum industry was saying there was no point in providing lead-free fuel because the car manufacturers do not demand it, and the car manufacturers were saying there was no point in supplying cars to run on lead-free petrol because the petroleum industry did not supply it.)

Rolls Royce wrote to say 'I can assure you that we are already producing cars which are designed to use lead-free petrol'.

Talbot were more forthcoming than they had been in reply to my earlier letter. However, their spokesman stated. . . .

> As a parent myself, I can entirely understand the reasons for your concern. However, I feel that you are, like many others, the innocent victim of a high-pressure publicity campaign dealing with an emotional subject. While it is true that the use of lead in petrol does lead to a very

small increase in the amount of lead in the atmosphere, the majority of this in fact comes from other sources which surround us in both home and the office environment.

Thus this Talbot spokesman, unlike the BL spokesman, did feel 'qualified' to comment on the health issue. How he could say that lead in petrol caused a 'very small increase in the amount of lead in the atmosphere' when it is accepted by all other parties in the controversy that lead in petrol contributes 90% of lead in the atmosphere, I really can't imagine. However, he then went on to say:

In spite of that, however, we, like all other vehicle manufacturers, are determined to do as much as we possibly can to eliminate this problem. As you state, there are some countries in which cars are operating on a lead-free petrol of the two-star octane. Unfortunately, in the interests of preservation of the world oil resources, the majority of cars in production today are designed to operate on four-star petrol, so giving the best possible fuel consumption, but equally requiring a very small amount of lead to achieve the fuel octane rating. Therefore, we are now working towards the dual objective of maintaining the fuel economy of our engines and reducing the octane demand of the engines, so that lead-free petrol can be used. Such an undertaking is of very large proportions, and it will be some time before the results of this work are available to the public. . . . Obviously for commercial and marketing reasons I am unable to give you either model names or dates for the introduction of these changes, since they will be coupled with other alterations to the cars, but I can assure you that they will take place.

This letter thus conceded that cars *could* be manufactured to run on lead-free petrol without the energy and other penalties that both industries had always maintained. Vauxhall also held out some hope in their letter to Mrs. Savery:

Our parent organisation, General Motors, are in the forefront of automotive design, and you can rest assured that if legislation is introduced into this country which forces the petrol companies to manufacture lead-free petrol, then we as a company will be ready to meet that challenge.

Ford replied:

Our policy is to build vehicles to use the available fuels, and lead-free petrol is not presently available in Britain, nor anywhere else in Europe. As soon as it is available then we shall meet the demand by manufacturing vehicles to use such petrol.

(In other words, the catch-22 of this issue!)
Ford, however, concluded: 'Rest assured, should lead-free

petrol become available, then Ford cars constructed to run on it would also be available.' Altogether, then, the individual car manufacturers came out of the exchanges a great deal better than the petroleum industry had done.

Anthony Fraser, Director of the Society of Motor Manufacturers and Traders, however, clearly had a different view of his responsibilities. He wrote to *The Times* to admit 'that car engines can, of course, be made to run on lead-free petrol'. He then however went on to attempt to show that 'airborne lead contributes directly between 3 and 10%' of the body lead burden. And that 'I am happy to think that my grandchild and any other grandchildren I may have should grow up in the United Kingdom where the lead in petrol will from 1985 be at a 0.15 grams per litre level'.

On the surface, the car manufacturers appear to come out of this affair better than the petroleum industry. Whether their position is any more defensible, however, is questionable. First, while individual companies have maintained a reasonably respectable public relations position, like the oil companies they have relied on their association, the Society of Motor Manufacturers and Traders, to do the dirty work. One of the Society's representatives was quoted in *The Guardian* as describing the anti-lead campaign as 'loony'. Like the petroleum companies, the car manufacturers have been happy to let Associated Octel 'front' the campaign for lead in petrol. Like the petroleum industry, the car manufacturers have been united in refusing to acknowledge responsibility for public health, refusing to concede the evidence of risk, and doggedly pursuing an industrial practice in the face of widespread public concern with no sign of conscience.

The Scientists
Given a controversy that is riddled with vested interests, how do you or I sort out fact from fiction? How do we decide whether lead in petrol causes ill effects or not?

Ideally we should be able to turn to science. Indeed, the importance of the scientific contribution to decision-making was plausibly argued by an 'environmental scientist' from the Rio Tinto

---

'We believe that the issue of industrial sponsorship . . . in many circumstances is a matter worthy of public attention. We and others have noticed that the nature of sponsorship is highly correlated with the conclusions about toxicity of lead.' *Herbert L. Needleman, Joseph Verducci, The Lancet, September 11, 1982.*

Zinc Corporation at a seminar in London in 1982. He argued that policy should be determined on the basis of the scientific consensus wherever possible. Less attention should be paid to 'legislating over' gaps in the scientific data base and much more to filling the deficiencies by appropriate research. The prime influence in standard setting should rest with the involved professionals. This scientist, A. K. Barbour, lamented the fact that 'regulators are greatly impressed – perhaps over-impressed – by the use of research workers operating in universities and other non-industrial laboratories. Indeed, so far as the European Commission is concerned, it seems to be almost impossible for industrial scientists to play a significant role . . . and yet they often have more detailed knowledge of the subject than anyone else'.

> The major influence in setting environmental performance criteria should revert to technical specialists having close practical experience of the subject under review and the views of specialists in industry – scientific – engineering and medical – should be taken seriously and not just dismissed as unprofessionally biased. . . . We must all embark on a programme to re-establish the credibility of industrial scientists, and medical people – and some regulatory agencies – in the eyes of the media.

I quote his remarks because I think it proper that this viewpoint should be acknowledged. I also accept without reservation that there should be a considerable scientific input into any decision-making process where it is relevant, and that where a scientific consensus is achieved it should be given considerable weight. However, I depart from him on two basic points:

First, the *extent* that decisions should be based upon the scientific input.

Second, the influence of industrial scientists.

Even the majority of scientists would accept that the decision on lead in petrol should not be left to them. Apart from the fact that they are divided themselves, and we would thus have to choose who to believe, this is one of those areas where science seems unable to be definite. In its purest form, science is a permanent search, non-stop revision, with a capacity to complicate and delay that can, when it comes down to the protection or otherwise of public health, sacrifice generations to research. Unfortunately, this is sometimes only too useful to the politicians; as a former Secretary of the US Academy of Science once said:

> It is a simple scientific fact that we can never know all we would like to know to assess the hazards of lead or any other toxic substance. It is an

unfortunate political fact that those with an economic stake in the outcome will exploit the limitations of science to delay, and if possible, prevent the social choices that can remove or ameliorate the probable hazards.

We have seen evidence of this in Britain during the last few years. No matter how much the medical evidence of health risk from lead has grown, the politicians have demanded more and more. Each study that purports to challenge the case for action is greeted with enthusiasm; each study that supports action is hyper-sensitively challenged. The inability of the scientists themselves to reach accord has played into the hands of the polluters. It is always disturbing to see medical authorities prepared to delay action in highly sensitive areas while they conduct further research and then further research, (often, it has to be said, to their own considerable financial benefit). Unfortunately, it is not merely the fallibility of science itself that we have to consider at this point, but also the fallibility of scientists. Scientists are no different from any other form of human life – there are able and clever scientists, and there are incompetent scientists; there are idealistic scientists and self-centred scientists; there are honest scientists and probably there are dishonest scientists. The best scientists would no doubt say that the worst were not scientists at all, but unfortunately they are presented to you and I as scientists. The best scientists, no doubt blinded by their own idealism and an almost touching innocence, take offence at the suggestion that scientists can be other than neutral, arguing they are always open to the impact of fresh evidence. This implies that they are a breed apart when it comes to fundamental human reactions – that they are not affected by material opportunities, the quest for fame, or pride. In circumstances where a scientist has abandoned, deliberately or otherwise, accepted standards of his profession, he may have ceased to be scientific, but he continues to have a scientific function, act as if he were a scientist and be treated as if he were a scientist.

It has also struck me forcibly during the lead in petrol debate that many scientists believe that their independence and integrity can be taken for granted just because they are scientists. But why should it be? It is of far greater importance that when it comes to matters of public controversy, justice is not only done but seen to be done.

If there is a question-mark over the neutrality of the scientist on a particular issue, his views on that particular issue have to be treated with reservations. This should not be seen as 'writing him off' scientifically. It simply means that there are a sufficient number of scientists of whom the question *cannot* be raised to make it unnecessary to prejudice the non-scientific response to scientific work by appointing to carry it out anyone who is perceived, rightly or wrongly, to have an in-built bias towards a given conclusion.

The environmental scientist quoted above was indignant because industrial scientists were, in his view, not given sufficient credence. But how can they really expect to be? As Dr. Clair Patterson has stated:

> In recent decades many fields in science have been invaded and taken over by industrial engineers and technologists, and science as a social institution has failed to respond to this challenge. Today engineering research and developmental activities greatly outnumber those of science, and are subtly blended with them. . . . Furthermore, sophisticated instruments are used by large numbers of engineers and technologists, masquerading as scientists, to gather data, promulgate sophistries and outnumber scientists in some areas such as environmental lead, so as to bury by sheer mass, questionable, erroneous, inaccurate data, and render ineffectual the tiny amount of correct scientific knowledge obtained by competent scientists in those fields.

What for instance do we make of the 'scientists' hired by companies like Associated Octel? If just one of them, just once, looked at the evidence and concluded that the company's product caused a health hazard, it just might be possible for the company to claim there was room within its ranks for objectivity. But, of course, that has never been the case. Their scientists attend the conferences, read the literature, work in laboratories, but always reach the opposite conclusions to the critics of their industry. So why do they undertake these activities? Are we really expected to believe that it is in the quest of truth? Is that why these companies pay them their salaries, send them all over the world to give lectures, publish their papers, and finance their work? Or is their responsibility really to find the escape route for industry? Is it not obvious that these industries would simply not hire anyone whose work to date, or opinions, were likely to challenge the industry's product?

When it comes to the lead-in-petrol issue in Britain, the record speaks for itself: not one doctor or scientist employed by Associated Octel, the petroleum industry, or the car-manufacturing industry, has ever done other than deny the health hazard, belittle the contribution of petrol lead to body lead burdens, and generally strengthen the industrial defence of the status quo. There is no exception. All the evidence of health hazard, and all the evidence of association between body lead burdens and petrol lead, have had to come from non-industrial scientists.

Then we come to the tricky question of scientists who are not employed directly by industry, but whose research activities are subsidised by industry or paid for entirely by industry, or who earn fees as advisers to industry. There is, of course, no reason why scientists should not be funded in this way. But, irrespective of whether or not this funding affects their objectivity, there can be little question that in the minds of those concerned about a particular related problem, their independence or openness of mind must at least be questionable? The extent that scientists have felt it necessary to protest at the links between industry and the contributions of some scientists on the lead and health question is well illustrated by the following letter to *the Lancet*, March 29, 1975:

Blood-Lead Levels, Behaviour, and Intelligence

Sir, – Dr McCabe's letter (Oct. 12, p. 896) criticising the Center for Disease Control's report of psychological deficit in children appears to be an exception to an observation we and others have made. . . .

We could find no statement, report, or study by an industry-sponsored scientist, whether in-house grantee, or academic consultant, which frankly acknowledges that low-level exposure is hazardous. Those reports of toxicity due to low-level lead exposure, on the other hand, tend to come from departments of public health, paediatrics, or environmental science. This observation appears well supported by the recent literature and by views expressed at three major meetings.

The association between nature of sponsorship and position on low-level lead toxicity appears challenged by Dr. McCabe's letter. Dr. McCabe cited his affiliation to an academic department of paediatrics in Wisconsin, but argued that low-level-lead effects have not been demonstrated. We find, however, that his text was first published almost verbatim as an International Lead Zinc Research Organisation In-House Report, dated July 16, 1974. In that report, the fact sheet lists him as 'Edward McCabe, Pediatric Consultant, ILZRO (International Lead Zinc Research Organisation)'.

It is not our interest to question Dr. McCabe's intent. That the lead industry supports research on the health effects of its products, and hires medical consultant for opinions, seems only proper. That these consultants acknowledge industry support when entering industry-sponsored comment into the scientific arena, seems to us not only proper, but obligatory.

Harvard Medical School, and Children's
   Hospital Medical Center   HERBERT L. NEEDLEMAN
Case Western Reserve University   SAMUEL EPSTEIN
University of Illinois, School of Public
   Health   BERTRAM CARNOW
Harvard Medical School   JOHN SCANLON
Hospital for Sick Children, Toronto   DAVID PARKINSON
Industrial Union Department, AFL-CIO   SHELDON SAMUELS
Oil, Chemistry and Atomic Workers   ANTHONY MAZZOCHI
State University of New York,
   Downstate   OLIVER DAVID

Then there are other scientists who have not only carried out research in a given area, but committed themselves to a position so consistently and forcefully that an admission of error or retraction, or change of position, would be more than embarrassing and could possibly create some lack of confidence in them within their field. Once more, I have no doubt there are many honourable scientists who would admit error. But how many? The honourable scientist would say that I put too much emphasis on the human beings and not enough on the nature of science. They would say that bad science always shows up in the end. They would say that taken overall the world of science is an honourable one and will not let humanity down. Unfortunately, in their innocence, they fail to see how industry and politicians can use some scientists to their advantage.

In the lead-in-petrol debate in Britain, four 'independent' scientists stand out as being most frequently cited by industry. They are Professor Patrick Lawther, Dr. Donald Barltrop, Dr. Tony Waldron, and Professor Barbara Clayton, all of them members of the DHSS working party, chaired by Lawther. As I have already commented, close scrutiny of the record of the debate shows that Lawther's Medical Research Council Air Pollution Unit consistently claimed to produce evidence that there was no serious cause for concern from airborne lead. In a 1980 article in *The Ecologist*, Nick Kollerstrom who had assisted Lawther for a number of years, stated:

> Professor Lawther, Chairman of the working party, was formerly Director of the MRC Research Unit. It is not unfair to point out that in that capacity he could always be relied upon to give assurance that existing levels of air pollutants were no danger to public health. . . . Such an expert was very valuable, and therefore, some would say, clearly the wrong person to ask to form this working party.

The real criticism of Lawther extends beyond the fact that he produced a bad report; it is that he at no stage after its publication sought to prevent its misuse by the defenders of lead in petrol, and at no stage sought to either clarify questions raised by Rutter or to contradict them. As the debate hotted up in 1982 he actually claimed that when his report recommended lead in petrol should be progressively reduced, it meant reduced to nil. I publicly challenged him to clarify that position once and for all by writing a letter to *The Times* stating that it was his and the Committee's view that lead should be phased out of petrol altogether. This would have made it impossible for Octel and the other industries to any longer quote Lawther in their defence. Lawther would not do it. As the controversy raged around him and his report, he would raise his head about the barricades occasionally, sometimes tossing out a remark that appeared to be supportive of the CLEAR case, and sometimes making a remark that further confused the issue.

In view of the use being made of his report, Lawther had a responsibility to clarify exactly what he believed it intended to say but he would not do so. His contribution to the reduction of other forms of pollution, particularly in London, had hitherto been commendable. It gives myself and CLEAR no pleasure to have to criticise his handling of the lead pollution issue. The record, however, speaks for itself.

Professor Barbara Clayton is another who over a number of years has published a considerable number of comments, papers, and studies, and consistently declined to acknowledge ill-effects from lead at low levels. She was one of the 'Great Ormond Street Four' who wrote the much-criticised critique of the Needleman and David studies, and is often quoted by Octel.

Dr. Tony Waldron is a special case, for in the early Seventies he worked closely with Dr. Robert Stephens in Birmingham, and then with Professor Bryce-Smith, and was perhaps the leading scientific campaigner on lead pollution and critic of the use of lead in petrol. In June 1974 Waldron signed with Bryce-Smith an article in *Chemistry in Britain*. It said:

> Present concern with lead as a toxic pollutant stems from the growing recognition that levels commonly present in city dwellers cause interference with the biosynthesis of haem and approach close to, and sometimes exceed, the threshold of potential clinical poisoning. There is also increasing evidence for a connection between childhood lead absorption and learning and behavioural disorders.

It also contained a section referring to the link between lead and delinquency and stated . . .

it is difficult to avoid the conclusion that toxic effects of lead on the human central nervous system may now be producing adverse *social* consequences of the most serious type (their emphasis).

On December 16, 1974, *The Birmingham Evening Mail* quoted Waldron as linking lead poisoning with offences such as football hooliganism. 'Such increasingly common offences as vandalism and football hooliganism are associated with hyperactivity', says Professor Waldron. 'And hyperactivity can be caused by high blood-lead levels. Lead levels in the blood of children living in cities is now at or above that at which behavioural disturbances are known to occur.' If this was a misreport, Waldron did not write to complain. However, by October 1979 in the *Journal of the Royal Society of Medicine* Waldron was saying:

> The conclusion that because a potentially toxic material can be detected it must be a hazard should be treated with the same objectivity as any other hypothesis, and we must not allow ourselves to be panicked into action which cannot be justified on scientific or medical grounds.

By then Waldron had completely changed his position, so much so that when Associated Octel were given the opportunity to nominate someone to appear on the BBC's *Today Programme* on their behalf, they nominated Waldron.

Perhaps the most controversial of all the scientists in the debate, however, is Dr. Donald Barltrop, a man who is particularly sensitive to reference to financial support he has received from the lead or anti-knock industry over the years. When Bryce-Smith led a discussion in BBC television's controversy series on 'Health hazards from lead pollution' in August 1971, Barltrop was one of five 'experts' who did battle with him. After *The Times* had published criticism of the performance of these 'experts' the following paragraph appeared in *The Times* in early September 1971:

> Dr. D. Barltrop of the Paediatric Unit at St. Mary's Hospital Medical School who took part on August 30 in a discussion on BBC 2 on the dangers of lead which was reviewed in *The Times* asks us to emphasise that he has no vested interest in lead.

Barltrop gave evidence for the petroleum industry in the Albery case in 1978. His affadavit said:

> From my knowledge and experience of the problem of childhood lead poisoning and exposure in all of the districts in which the plaintiffs reside, I can say that urban children are all exposed to lead from numerous sources but that by far the major part of their body lead burdens derive from the ingestion of foodstuffs and beverages and not from the inhalation of atmospheric lead.

(In no way did Barltrop indicate in his affidavit any recognition that atmospheric lead enters the body other than by inhalation; it seems incredible that a scientist who has studied lead would not be aware of the other ways whereby airborne lead reaches human beings.) He then went on to refer to different possibilities of exposure other than lead from petrol.

> I have read the affadavits of Eleanor Margaret Budden and Nicholas Albery (the parents) and can say that the behaviour attributed to their children is commonplace, and may be related to a wide variety of social and medical conditions and would not in itself, or indeed in conjunction with the results of the test on the plaintiff children indicate undue lead exposure. . . . I have read the particulars of claim and plaintiffs affidavits in all three actions. There are many claims in them which I consider to be without a scientific basis and contrary to general scientific and medical thinking in this field.

I wrote to Barltrop to ask him whether he had been paid a fee for this testimony and other such support for the industrial position. He refused to answer.

In March 1979 Barltrop gave evidence at a public enquiry into the building of the M25 motorway. The objectors were citing lead pollution as one of the many reasons why they did not wish the motorway to be built. His contributions included:

> As far as the question of lead from motor cars is concerned, as generally encountered in cities in parts of this country, I would agree with the statement that there is no evidence of a general health hazard, and I say this because the evidence so far is that the contribution of airborne lead to blood lead values is relatively small, particularly when compared to other sources of lead which are a very real hazard for children living in our cities.

Of Needleman (and other) studies:

> They show only association, there is as yet no evidence of dose response relationship.

(The opposite is in fact the case; the higher the lead level, the greater the behavioural problem Needleman found.)

> I think no evidence has been produced to show that there is in fact any deleterious effect at that level (20 ug/dl) in terms of health.

> There is no evidence that pervading levels of airborne lead in the environment in general constitutes a hazard.

> I find it very difficult to get a definition of this term sub-clinical and in a sense it is a misnomer because sub-clinical means something that

can't be detected clinically and if it can't be detected, then it isn't there . . . (Uproar from audience) . . . I think you can only argue that an effect is there if you can find it.

If you are asking me, do I think there is a hazard there within the limits which we have been discussing . . . then I cannot see that there is an identifiable risk in relation to the other sources which they are already exposed to at this moment.
(Inspector) I think you are saying there is no identifiable risk.
(Barltrop) This is what I am saying.

It is surely fair to say that given the needs of industry to produce supportive evidence for its position, it is more likely to purchase the expertise from those it knows to be sympathetic to its position, rather than the other way round. Thus, when the industries nominate someone to represent them, or employ someone to undertake research on their behalf, they are surely indicating their belief that these particular scientists have a confirmed view. If industries feel sufficiently confident that a scientist is likely to reach conclusions sympathetic to it because of that scientist's prior position, can members of the public be blamed if they also expect such a result? The position of Lawther, Clayton, Waldron, and Barltrop on the likelihood of health damage by lead in petrol was sufficiently well-known when the Lawther Committee was set up for the anti-lead movement to be entitled to feel uneasy, and the subsequent report justified this pessimism.

In my view, scientists cannot be assumed to be objective if there is every reason to believe that their attachment to established positions is such that it would require a disproportionate weight of evidence on the other side to change them. In the case of Waldron, he had made an extreme change from one position (that lead exposure was causing football hooliganism) to another (that it was 'of no more significance than a gnat farting in the Albert Hall'). For him to change his position once more and acknowledge that he was more likely to be correct in his earlier days would surely be an incredibly difficult reverse to make.

Those who were concerned about the impartiality and objectivity of the Lawther Committee and who were so deeply con-

'I think sir that perhaps there is no necessity for Dr. Barltrop to answer my questions. . . . I have listened to him for about six hours now and it seems to me that his position is so deeply entrenched and inflexible that nothing I, a mere layman, can ask, will possibly have any effect on his curiously defensive attitude.' *Objector at the M25 motorway enquiry.*

cerned about the issue, had every reason to be concerned. There were reasonable grounds for doubt as to whether the Committee would be objective. There were reasonable grounds for doubt as to whether some members of the Committee could approach the matter with an open mind. It is questionable whether two or three of its members should have been on it. Of more importance, an attempt should have been made to balance the Committee by at least one, if not two, members whom the petroleum industry had the same cause to fear as the anti-lead movement had the members of the Committee chosen.

What is even more disturbing is that Ministers are now putting their faith in a number of new studies into the health effects of lead. They so desperately need these studies to reinforce their view, and also to reinforce the Lawther report, that the anti-lead movement are understandably concerned that the key personalities involved, Clayton and Yule and Lansdown, were members of the Lawther Committee. They are effectively being asked to sit in judgement on their own findings. Not only is Clayton responsible for one of the studies, but she sits on the MRC Committee that makes judgements on the Yule and Lansdown study. Given that she is also on the Royal Commission, her power on this issue has become considerable. It is, of course, not my suggestion that anyone would alter the data, but as we have seen, data can be interpreted in different ways, and there is little question that Associated Octel and the other vested interests would rather have Barbara Clayton interpreting the data from her established viewpoint than, say, Professor Rutter. It would have made much more sense, in terms of reassuring public opinion, if neutral scientists had been employed for this exercise. CLEAR and the public as a whole can hardly be blamed if they fear a repeat performance of Lawther.

Why have I included scientists under the heading 'The Guilty Ones'? Because I believe on this issue the medical community has failed our children. It did so when it first devised the idea of putting lead in petrol and thus created the pollutant. It has done so by failing until very recent times to identify low level lead pollution as the problem. It has done so by allowing industrial scientists and those funded by industry to have too much unchallenged prominence in the debate. It has done so by failing to come up with a working party that everyone concerned with the issue would feel was balanced. And it has done so by demonstrating its capacity to delay.

That is why I say the decision on issues of this sort can never be left to the scientists who created the pollutant, who are divided on the issue, or who want to continue with research and more research, with successive generations of children as their guinea pigs. Science can and should and must have its say, but there has to come a moment when the evidence they produce is evaluated and common sense applied, the level of risk considered and a decision taken by the community as a whole. The decision is ours.

As a former President of the Conservation Society, Lord Avebury, has said:

> This is a political decision which cannot be left to the scientists alone. The scientists advise, and they differ in their opinions. Ultimately it is for each one of us to form a judgement on the evidence presented as to what degree of protection is needed. If we are forced to the conclusion that the health of future generations may be undermined, then it will be through the political process that remedies have to be sought.

The Politicians

It apparently serves Ministers to portray the CLEAR campaign and myself as unreasonable and extreme. In a letter to a Conservative MP on July 22, 1982 the man who coordinates policies on lead, Giles Shaw, at the DOE, described the activities of CLEAR as 'extremist pressure'. In fact (and in retrospect it was perhaps naïve) the launch of CLEAR was planned on the assumption that Ministers were prepared to be open-minded on the issue. At the launch I emphasised that the Conservatives had, with the reduction to 0.15 grams per litre, at least done more than other parties; our policy was at that stage not to condemn them for indifference to lead pollution but rather to encourage them to take their policy a stage further.

Indeed, a key factor in the CLEAR decision to accept the limit of 0.15 grams per litre for *existing* cars, albeit demanding that this happened earlier than 1985, was as we openly declared in our handbook, that 'we have made it unnecessary for any political party to defend its present position, for what we propose is not a reversal of present policy, but rather a further extension of it.' I even arranged to meet Giles Shaw a few days before the launch in order to brief him on the campaign. At that meeting I explained to him that CLEAR had no intention of attacking Ministers and intended to take a positive attitude to what had been done. In return for this I repeated my hope that Ministers would at least keep an open mind on the issue. Unfortunately, this did indeed prove to be over-optimistic.

Within hours of my meeting with Shaw the instructions went out: first, two DOE officials gate-crashed the launch press conference in order to report back to Whitehall where plans were already being laid to try to knock down the CLEAR campaign before it was on its feet. On the day of the launch Shaw together with Health Minister,

Kenneth Clarke, issued a dogmatic document to all MPs describing CLEAR's campaign as unrealistic. From the start they made it clear that a positive dialogue was impossible and they were prepared and even anxious for battle.

So much for any suggestion that CLEAR from the outset adopted a confrontational approach.

Whitehall then tried to coordinate its replies to anxious letters from MPs and parents. To illustrate the extent of this let me quote the activities of a civil servant by the name of R. G. Baker. On June 30, Baker wrote to a member of the public from Hounslow, Middlesex as follows:

> Your letter concentrates on lead in petrol, but the Government's policy is a comprehensive one and is directed to reducing human exposure to lead in the environment wherever practicable. Clearly it is overall exposure (from whatever source) that matters and we must look at all potential sources. That is why action on lead in water and food is so important as well. . . . To put the matter in perspective, our assessment of the evidence is that the typical city dweller probably now gets about 20% of his environmental lead intake from petrol containing the present 0.4 grams per litre – about 10% coming direct from the air and as much again indirectly through other pathways.

This letter was on *Department of Environment* paper. However, on June 21, 1982, a civil servant also called R. G. Baker had written on *Department of Transport* paper to a doctor in Plaistow, London. He stated:

> Your letter concentrates on lead in petrol, but the Government's policy is a comprehensive one and is directed to reducing human exposure to lead in the environment wherever practicable. Clearly it is overall exposure (from whatever source) that matters and we must look at all potential sources. That is why action on lead in water and food is so important as well. . . . To put the matter in perspective, our assessment of the evidence is that the typical city dweller probably now gets about 20% of his environmental lead intake from petrol containing the present 0.4 grams per litre – about 10% coming direct from the air and as much again indirectly through other pathways.

The same words.

On July 2, 1982, the same R. G. Baker (or presumably the same) still writing on *Department of Transport* paper to a member of the public in Camden, London, used exactly the same words. However, an R. G. Baker writing on DOE paper a couple of days before to a member of the public in St. Albans, Hertfordshire, also used the same words.

Baker is but one of a number of civil servants who are almost full-time employed answering letters from concerned members of the public and who too easily find fault with every piece of lead pollution evidence. They have been doing this for some years. For instance, in the mid-seventies there was an extraordinary letter by Dr. E. E. Simpson, Senior Principal Medical Officer, to the National Union of Teachers, stating 'It is the case that West Germany provides petrol with a lower lead content than does the rest of the Community, but this was done mainly with the object of producing engines for export to certain parts of the world where other pollution problems as well as lead in air exist.' This was disgracefully misleading. To begin with, the German reduction to 0.15 grams per litre would not meet the problem Simpson refers to; what he is concerned about is the effect of leaded petrol on catalytic converters, and only lead-free petrol is suitable for them, thus the reduction to 0.15 in Germany would not help at all. Second, the West German Economic Ministry in September 1978, confirmed that . . .

> The basis of the West German decision to enact legislation for lowering the lead content of petrol was the realisation that the concentration of lead compounds in automobile exhaust gases constitutes a health hazard to the population. Lead and its compounds have long been recognised everywhere as one of the most toxic elements in existence. The lead emissions of exhaust gases are particularly dangerous in this respect since they occur in the form of minute particles which reach the pulmonary tract in respired air.

In August 1981 a DOE civil servant wrote:

> To adopt the option of lead-free petrol would have to await the design of new engines, their production and the progressive replacement of existing engines as the latter came to the end of their useful lives. This would take many years; perhaps ten years for design and production. . . .

In December of that year the British Leyland Technical Director said in a letter:

> Assuming a change to low octane lead-free fuel (we could introduce cars able to run on lead-free petrol) in about five years and with a maintained octane number in about half this time.

In July 1982 I wrote to a DOE civil servant, F. Kendall, challenging letters he had been writing to members of the public. In particular I was concerned about his attempts to refute the import-ance of the NHANES 11 study from the United States and the Turin isotope study. He replied on the NHANES study:

The researchers have firmly refused to claim a cause-effect relationship between the production of petrol lead and the fall in blood-lead levels. . . . I understand that Dr. Annest himself made this point at your recent symposium.

On the Turin study he stated:

From what we know of atmospheric and petrol lead levels in Turin (potentially higher than in the UK) and local climatic conditions (frequently anticyclones trapping stagnant air, especially in summer), however, I should be surprised if the Ispra results were directly applicable to the UK.

I replied:

The fact of the matter is that you and your colleagues at the DOE and other Ministries are not in the least concerned with examining the evidence on the issues objectively, but look at every piece of evidence from the point of view of how you could possibly undermine it or question it. This is shown, for instance, by your selective quotations. For instance, you make the point that Annest 'firmly refused' to claim a cause-effect relationship between the reduction in petrol lead and the fall in blood-lead levels. It is true that he did not claim a cause-effect relationship, but to say that he 'firmly refused' creates a misleading impression. In fact, his final words were 'The *striking similarity* between the decrease in the use of lead in the production of petrol, and the drop in mean blood-lead levels, is suggestive that lead entering the atmosphere from the combustion of leaded petrol can contribute *significantly* to the level of lead in human beings'.

On Kendall's comments on the Turin experiment I pointed out:

You once more try to suggest that it is not applicable to the UK by an almost pathetic search for any explanation but the obvious. Whether or not there are 'frequent anticyclones trapping stagnant air' has no bearing on the fact that this was the area carefully chosen by the EEC for these studies and the results happen to be inconvenient for the DOE and British policy.

What has been even more extraordinary has been the behaviour of Tory Ministers such as Mr. Kenneth Clarke. Within two months of taking office, Kenneth Clarke, then Parliamentary Under Secretary for Transport, was taking a complacent line on lead in petrol. When Jeff Rooker, responding to a story in the *Birmingham Post* that research with 379 pre-school youngsters had indicated that one in 15 had higher lead levels in their blood than EEC limits (themselves too high), Clarke replied that he saw 'no justification' for speeding up the reduction to 0.40 by January 1981. Rooker described the reply as 'unbelievably smug and complacent'.

Any hope that Clarke would look at the subject afresh when he became Minister of Health was somewhat diminished from March 12, 1982, when *The Times* reported that he spent most of his first week 'closeted with his civil servants'. He went on 'I am very conscious I have an enormous amount to learn but when I went to the Department of Transport I knew very little about that either. But, given good civil servants, I didn't find it a big handicap'. The civil servants must have loved that.

In reply to a question in the House of Commons on May 20, 1982, Clarke said:

I have now had an opportunity to study the British Medical Association's evidence to the Royal Commission on Environmental Pollution. It is a balanced document reaching similar conclusions to those reached a year ago by the Government following publication of the report by the DHSS working party on Lead and Health, chaired by Professor Patrick Lawther. I welcome it as reinforcing the Government's view of the need for a series of measures based on the recommendations of that report. We announced a programme in May last year and nothing in this report reduces our confidence in the desirability of that programme.

I understand that in the course of a careful summing up of the recent CLEAR symposium, Professor Michael Rutter, who was a member of the Working Party, expressed the personal view that it would be prudent to remove lead entirely from petrol. He however acknowledged the uncertainty of the medical evidence on the effects of very low levels of lead in the body.

I wrote to Clarke in reply:

Your parliamentary answer to Neville Trotter, MP (May 20), misled the House and the nation. In its cynicism it largely explains why so many people are disillusioned with politicians.

Firstly, you refer to the British Medical Association's evidence to the Royal Commission on Environmental Pollution as 'reaching similar conclusions to those reached a year ago by the Government following publication of the report of the DHSS Working Party on Lead and Health. . . . I welcome it as reinforcing the Government's view of the need for a series of measures based on the recommendations of that report.'

This is a complete distortion of the BMA's evidence. First, the Lawther report and *the Government have stood on a safety level of 35 ug/dl*. The BMA contradicts this saying 'There is evidence that *children who have body burdens of lead lower than that indicated by 30 ug/dl may be at risk*. Associations have been demonstrated between impairment and mental functioning and lead levels below the range previously considered harmful.'

Second, whereas the Government has continued to take the view that a reduction of 0.15 grams per litre is adequate, and that *eliminating lead from petrol would in any case only affect about 10–20% of the body lead burden*, the BMA specifically says 'taking into account all the available evidence it would appear that the elimination of lead from petrol would reduce considerably the concentration of lead in the atmosphere. This in turn would produce a reduction in the burden of lead absorbed by individuals. For those individuals already exposed to higher than average concentrations of atmospheric lead, *the body burden might be reduced by as much as one third.*'

This is a contradiction of both the Lawther and the Government position.

I now refer to your outrageous misrepresentation of the summing-up of the CLEAR symposium by Professor Michael Rutter. While acknowledging that he took the view that it would be prudent to remove lead entirely from petrol, you seek to suggest that he did so without enthusiasm by continuing '*He however acknowledged the uncertainty of the medical evidence* on the effects of very low levels of lead in the body'.

A true reflection can be gained from the following quotations from Professor Rutter:

'We cannot be sure that the effects of lead are real, but the balance of evidence suggests they are. . . . *It is evident that the best and most recent studies have failed to disprove the hypothesis that low level lead exposure leads to psychological impairment. . . . The implication is that it would be both safer in practice, and scientifically more appropriate, to act as if the hypothesis were true, rather than continue to act as if it were not true.*

The risk seems to be substantially more than a trivial one and, at least in some individuals, the effects are likely to be of practical importance in causing impairment of functioning. The implication is that *we now know enough to warrant taking such public health action as* are *likely to reduce lead pollution in the environment. . . . The removal of lead from petrol would seem to be one of those worthwhile public health actions. . . .* In my view, the reduction of lead in petrol to an intermediate level is an unacceptable compromise without clear advantages and with definite disadvantages.'

There is simply no point of contact between the message of Professor Michael Rutter, who after all was a member of the Lawther Committee, and the Government.

On July 7, I had cause to write to Clarke once more:

We have already had cause to complain about your misquotation of authorities on lead pollution and health; I am afraid that I once more have cause to complain about the cynicism and dishonesty of a Parliamentary answer, this time your answer to Alf Dubs on July 7 when you stated that 'there is no convincing evidence that harm is caused at blood-lead levels below 35 ug/dl.

Firstly, you once more dishonestly imply that the British Medical Association's evidence to the Royal Commission on Environmental Pollution was supportive of your position. This is not so. . . . No doubt the BMA were more convinced than you appear to be of the importance of the Yule and Lansdown pilot study confirming the Needleman study in the United States – i.e. a finding of an average IQ deficit of seven points among children at 13 ug/dl and above.

The real position is not that you know of no convincing evidence, but that no evidence will convince you.

Let's look at some other Ministerial decisions or distortions:

> In our view, none of the recent evidence adds significantly to the information available to us when we made the decision . . . announced last May. (Giles Shaw, 25/3/82; Lynda Chalker 22/4/82)

Incorrect: there have been a number of major items of evidence associating lead with neurological dysfunction since Ministers took their decision on the basis of the Lawther Committee report and none are consistent with Lawther's conclusions. That is why Rutter, reviewing the up-to-date evidence, stated: 'The best of the most recent studies indeed fail to disprove the hypothesis that low level lead exposure leads to psychological impairment.' That is why the BMA decided that 'At first there was some doubt about the validity of these studies but it is now generally accepted that the association is real.'

> Taken as a whole, the results (of an EEC screening of blood-lead levels) reinforce the Government's view that levels of lead pollution in the environment give no cause for alarm. (Giles Shaw 30/6/82)

Incorrect: the studies indicate few children with blood-lead levels over 35 ug/dl. Good news – if that was a safe level. But as I have made clear, this threshold is at least three times too high.

> For most people lead from petrol contributes directly only a small proportion of their total intake of lead – less than 10% on average, possibly as much as 20% in the case of people who live and work close to a heavily trafficked road. (Giles Shaw 23/12/81)

> A typical town dweller probably gets about 20% of his environmental lead intake from petrol – about 10% directly from the air, and about 10% indirectly through other pathways. (Giles Shaw 25/3/82)

Contradiction: Assuming 'average' to mean 'typical', Shaw doubled his estimate of the average/typical lead intake from petrol in only three months. Even so, he was underestimating the petrol contribution to body lead burdens by at least 100% and probably more.

> Most people's lead intake comes not from petrol but from food. (Giles Shaw 14/4/82)

> Clearly it is overall exposure – from whatever source – that matters – we must look at all potential sources. That is why action on lead in water and food is important as well. (Lynda Chalker 17/5/82)

Deception: By then both these Ministers knew only too well that food was not a *source* of lead pollution, but a *route*. This is typical of the way the Ministers shuffle the cards and mislead people who have not studied the matter.

> We should of course take into account any recommendations made to us by the Royal Commission on Environmental Pollution who have recently embarked on a study of lead in the environment. (Lynda Chalker 22/4/82)

Misleading: The Royal Commission had excluded a review of the health issue and thus its findings would be irrelevant to the fundamental issue – should lead be banned from petrol because of the health hazard? Naturally Ministers were only too happy to encourage anticipation of the Commission whose objectives suggest a whitewash.

> We are reducing the lead level by over 60% in the four years ending in 1985. (Lynda Chalker 16/6/82)

Completely untrue: This implies lead intake will be considerably less during the following four years and reduced by 60% by the end of 1985. In fact, the petroleum companies have to reduce the lead levels by the *end* of 1985 and few have even begun to take the necessary steps. Lead levels would remain the same for nearly all of that four years.

> Lead-free petrol . . . will not really be an option for the vast bulk of cars that will be on our roads into the 1990s. Indeed probably no more than 10% of the 15 million petrol-driven vehicles currently on our roads could use it. (Hamish Gray 17/5/82)

Prevaricative: A classic Ministerial manoeuvre is to decline to reject a non-existent proposal to avoid facing a real one. Few have asked that lead-free petrol should be introduced for existing cars, rather that lead levels should be reduced for them whilst a date should be fixed for the phasing out of lead in petrol *in new cars*. Ministers know this but like to confuse the issue by talking about problems with existing cars.

The following correspondence concerning Sir George Young indicates the extent that Ministers will go to to try and mislead the public. On July 31 he wrote to a constituent:

> Your quotation from the BMA about 'levels of exposure previously considered safe' refers to a blood-lead level of 80 micrograms per 100 millilitres – a level long recognised as potentially dangerous – and *not* to 35 ug/100ml.

Fortunately the constituent forwarded the letter to me. I was able to reply, copying the letter to Young:

> Sir George Young is incorrect. There can be no question as to what the BMA were referring to if you take the relevant paragraphs: 'Several authorities . . . have prescribed a lead level of 35 ug/dl (30 ug/dl for children) or above as indicating an unacceptable level of lead exposure. Surveys in the UK show that the majority of the population has levels below this. Lead hot-spots have been identified where a few individuals exceed this level.'
>
> 'However, there is evidence that children who have body burdens of lead lower than indicated by 30 ug/dl may be at risk. Associations have been demonstrated between impairment in mental functioning and lead levels below the range previously considered harmful. At first there was some doubt about the validity of these studies but it is now generally accepted that the association is real.'
>
> This crucial section of their report – the section that CLEAR quotes – is clearly referring to 35 and 30 ug/dl and below.
>
> However, even the subsequent quote later that 'on the basis of the evidence which it has received, the BMA considers that lead is capable of causing harm at levels of exposure previously considered safe' goes on to say 'i.e. levels indicated by lead between 30 ug/dl–80 ug/dl'.
>
> Sir George Young misrepresents this to say that 'It refers to a blood-lead level of 80 ug/100ml'.
>
> This is a completely dishonest representation by any standards and I am appalled that he should be responsible for it.

Young was clearly sufficiently embarrassed by this to write once more to the constituent:

> First may I apologise unreservedly? As you rightly point out, the BMA piece about levels of exposure previously considered safe referred to a range between 30–80 ug/dl, not as I said, simply to 80 ug/dl. I have received a copy of Mr. Wilson's letter to you making rather more of a meal of an accidental slip-up than seems warranted.

So there it is. 'An accidental slip-up'. Yet Young had chosen his words with care and actually underlined *not* to 35 ug/100ml.

By now correcting Ministers' distortions was becoming an exhausting business. Nor was it confined to the Commons. In the

House of Lords on March 29, 1982, The Earl of Avon misled the House by suggesting that the only reason for eliminating lead from petrol in the United States and Japan was to protect catalytic converters. 'There is plenty of evidence from both countries that health factors were also of the utmost importance,' I wrote to him and then detailed the evidence I have already covered in this book. Lord Avon had to reply:

> On re-reading the answers to supplementary questions in Hansard, I agree that I was too categorical as regards the reasons for the policies that have been adopted in the USA, Japan, and Australia. . . . I agree that they, like us, have always wanted to reduce total lead emissions because of the possible hazard to health.

I replied:

> Thank you for your letter of April 30 to acknowledge that you misinformed the House. I shall look forward to reading in Hansard of your correction of that misinformation.

It never was corrected. Nor was the misleading of the public restricted to Ministers.

On April 1, 1982, Sir Angus Maude MP, former Cabinet Minister responsible for promoting the image of the Government, wrote to a constituent in Stratford on Avon to say:

> As you say, the Government is taking the question of lead in petrol very seriously, and hopes to progress towards lead-free petrol as quickly as possible.

Unfortunately untrue!

What does all this add up to? Of course it is reasonable for Ministers to defend their policies, especially if they believe them. If they had entered into a fair and open-minded dialogue with CLEAR and its many supporting organisations, and if they had indicated a genuine desire to look at the evidence objectively, it would be possible to accept that they genuinely believe that they were following the correct course. But there is plenty of evidence that they are making no attempt to be open-minded or to keep pace with the developing debate. They continue to repeatedly cite the Lawther report, even though they themselves have abandoned at least three of its key conclusions. They selectively quote from documents and often misquote from them. They approach every new study or piece of evidence in a hyper-critical way, they contradict each other, they demand conclusive evidence even whilst being aware that it is unobtainable, and they make no attempt to answer criticisms or questions directly.

On each occasion I have written to a Minister making a number of detailed points and raising detailed questions, I have received a short, prevaricative, complacent answer. They deal arrogantly with the concern of members of the public by sending the same letter to everyone, adapting it occasionally after the correspondence has been forwarded to CLEAR and they realise they can no longer get away with a particular argument.

You may say, why be surprised? What do you expect of politicians? My answer would be that it is one thing to adopt debating tactics at election time, or in ultra-political exchanges in the House of Commons, and another to adopt them in an all-out attempt to allay concern about environmental pollution and to avoid their responsibilities for the protection of public health.

One cannot but wonder whether they would have ever been in a position where they needed to defend the reduction to 0.15 grams per litre if the House of Commons had the information in their possession that Tom King had when he announced the reduction – that the petroleum industry were ready and willing to move towards lead-free petrol, and that the nation's Chief Medical Officer of Health had urged that such action be taken. The nation's legislators were entitled to that knowledge. The fact that when the Yellowlees letter was eventually published, the leaders of both the Labour and Liberal Parties, Michael Foot and David Steel, felt provoked to question the Prime Minister on this subject, indicates what their reaction would have been in May 1981 had the House been properly briefed. But it was not. The cover-up began then and it continues to this day.

8.
Towards lead free petrol

LEAD IS not a natural component of petrol. There is no lead in petrol. All that is necessary to produce lead-free petrol is not to add lead. It is as simple as that.

The real problem, then, is how to produce cars that will operate effectively on unleaded petrol. As the Japanese have conclusively proven, this is not difficult. Indeed, the absurdity of the British position is that the Japanese, having manufactured their cars to run on lead-free petrol to protect their own children, have to adapt them for the British market so that, like British cars, they can pollute the air. (At least one Honda model will produce 59 miles per gallon on unleaded petrol in Japan, but after adaptation for the British market, can only produce 47 miles per gallon on leaded fuel – yet we are told leaded petrol is best for fuel economy!)

The Japanese decided in 1970 that lead was an unacceptable exhaust emission and since February 1976 all regular petrol has been required to be lead-free and new cars have been required to run on it. Note the following:

(1)   The Japanese Consumer's Association reports that 92 octane lead-free petrol was produced 'without raising the retail price at gas stations'.

(2)   Premium petrol with lead was retained for existing cars, but by the end of 1982 less than 4% of petrol produced in Japan was 'premium', for the Japanese found that low octane lead-free petrol did *not* lead to increased fuel consumption or reduced car efficiency as predicted, and therefore virtually abandoned 'premium' altogether.

(3)   The move to lead-free petrol has not hindered the Japanese car manufacturing industry; on the contrary, the main threat to the European car manufacturing industry in the Eighties comes not from the threat of lead-free petrol but from Japanese imports.

As explained in chapter one, the Americans also began to phase lead out of petrol in 1975. Major petrol retailers were required by law to sell at least one grade of unleaded petrol (containing no more than 0.013 grams per litre) and car manufacturers required to make cars to run on lead-free petrol. At the same time the lead permitted in leaded petrol for old cars was to be phased down over a five year period from 0.45 grams per litre to 0.13 grams per litres by 1980. American cars too, are now manufactured to run on low octane petrol.

It is one of the further ironies of the situation that in order to export British cars for the American and Japanese markets, the British manufacturers have had to design cars and manufacture them to run on lead-free petrol. Thus, they are in the opposite position to Japanese and American manufacturers in that they are adapting cars to protect Japanese and American children whilst refusing to offer the same protection to children in their own country.

Australia is the third country dedicated to lead-free petrol. It will be introduced there in 1985. A major influence there has been the work of Professor Lloyd Smythe and colleagues. They tested children in schools in four different parts of Sydney, one in an industrial area with heavy traffic, one near a busy traffic intersection, and two on the outer fringe of the suburban area. They carefully measured the lead content in air at these localities, took samples of blood, hair and urine of children to analyse the lead and asked teachers to evaluate classroom performance and behaviour. They declared their results showed:

> Similar trends to specific behaviour effects of lead now being reported from overseas studies. . . . Whenever anti-social or delinquent children were encountered, they had raised lead levels.

While Australia intends to follow the Japanese and Americans and introduce catalytic converters to control other emissions, the Australians have made it very clear that the fundamental reason for the control of lead in petrol was to protect the public from its adverse effects. The fact that lead damages catalytic converters was a secondary consideration.

Why Lead in Petrol?

The function of lead in petrol was well described in a joint BEUC/EEB discussion document in 1982:

> The efficiency of a car engine depends on the compression ratio. In general the higher the compression ratio, the lower the fuel consumption. Increasing the compression ratio is, however, limited by combustion problems, that manifest themselves as 'knocking' or 'pinking'. The onset of knocking can be prevented or delayed by a good design of cylinder heads and by the use of fuels with a high anti-knock rating . . . the anti-knock characteristics of petrols (are reflected in an octane number).

To determine the octane number, two tests are used. The first simulates accelerating from low speed. The octane number found under these conditions is called the research octane number or RON. 'Accelerating knock' – if it occurs – is being heard by the driver. The second test simulates the driving conditions at high and constant speed. The corresponding octane number is called motor octane number or MON. Knocking under these circumstances is called 'high speed knock' and will not be heard by the driver owing to road and wind noise. If it continues for a long time, however, it can damage the engine. The difference between the two octane numbers is called sensitivity. When petrol is marketed normally only the research octane number is stated. In the 1920s it was discovered that certain organic lead compounds could improve the octane rating of petrol. For a long time only tetraethyl lead (TEL) was used to increase the octane rating. In the course of developing petrol with increased high octane numbers, however, it was found that in some cases tetramethyl lead (TML) offered greater advantages. The alkyl lead compounds tetraethyl lead and tetramethyl lead are both used in current motor fuels.

In cars with unhardened valve seats lead compounds also provide protection against valve seat wear, because lead acts as a lubricant.

The British Department of Transport says of leaded petrol:

This makes the petrol suitable for use in high compression engines which are more efficient than their low compression equivalents. If high compression engines are run on petrol with insufficient octane rating 'knocking' – a form of uncontrolled combustion – results, and this can cause serious damage. Lead also acts as a valve seat lubricant and engines designed to take advantage of this characteristic will be damaged if operated on lead-free fuel, whether or not it is of the correct octane rating.

This is a typical Whitehall over-simplification. First, the claim that high compression engines 'are more efficient' begs a number of questions. For instance, what, in terms of a motor car, is efficiency? Is it miles per gallon? If so, this has been no problem for the Americans and the Japanese. Is it speed? Low compression cars will more than meet the speed limits on European roads. Is it acceleration? Few drivers will have their lives drastically affected if their cars leave a stationary position a fraction of a second slower than they would with a high compression engine. The fact is, that Americans with their huge eight-lane highways and vast open spaces and big cars find low compression engines satisfactory.

Second, when the DOT talks about lead acting as a 'valve seat lubricant for engines designed to take advantage of the characteristic', what they really mean is for engines designed to be produced on the cheap. The fact is that for only a few more pence British cars could be produced with hardened valve seats, as some already are, and as they are in Japan, and the problem would be solved.

What has actually been happening is that the petroleum and motor car industry have been marketing unnecessarily high performance. With the petroleum companies it was 'the tiger in your tank'. Motorists liked the idea that they were buying a bit of extra power. The fact that they already had the power they needed for the permissible speed limits escaped them. Likewise, car manufacturers make much of the 'top speed' their car will travel. The fact that their 'top speed' is anywhere from 20–40 miles above the permitted speed limit should make their ads irrelevant. They are, in effect, manufacturing a product for an illicit market – car owners who exceed the speed limit. If their technology was concentrated on producing the best possible results, with maximum road safety and minimum pollution, at 70 miles per hour, they could well be more competitive with the Japanese.

Britain's Options
Britain, basically, has three options:

Firstly, it can introduce low octane (92 RON or 2-star) petrol into all retail outlets. New cars would be required to be manufactured to use it. This course is favoured by the petroleum industry who say they can produce 92-octane lead-free petrol quickly and at little cost. Indeed, a senior BP executive said in 1982 that it could be produced within a few months for an extra penny a gallon. The disadvantages are twofold: first, the major cost would be borne by Britain's ailing car manufacturing industry. This would need to produce cars able to operate efficiently on 92 octane fuel. Second, it is possible that at least half the existing cars on the road would not operate efficiently on low octane fuel, and thus it would be necessary to maintain a leaded high-octane (4-star) and phase the lead out over a generation of cars, delaying the elimination of this pollution. This route has been chosen by the three countries so far dedicated to lead-free petrol, America, Japan, and Australia, and is the route favoured by the BEUC–EEB European campaign. Whether or not they have fully investigated the matter, Britain's car manufacturers also seem to imply in all they say that they believe this to be the only realistic route to lead-free petrol.

The second option is that car manufacturers could produce cars with very minor modification but that all retail outlets would be supplied with high-octane lead-free fuel. The cost would now be minimal to the car manufacturing industry, the burden being carried by the petroleum industry. This industry says the cost of modifying refining processes would be prohibitive and there would be a heavy energy penalty.

The third option is to explore a variety of other alternatives, from the replacement of lead with other additives intended to achieve the same purpose, such as MTBE, to the greater use of LPG or diesel, or the implementation of lead filters.

MTBE is methyl tertiary butyl ether. A Scottish consortium, Highland Hydrocarbons, has been hoping to build a plant to produce this in Scotland despite obstacles placed in its path by Whitehall. It would produce 500,000 tons a year. The Davey Design Engineering Group, developers of the technology, claimed in the *Financial Times* in May 1981 that two 500,000 tons a year plants would create enough petrol additive to meet Britain's entire octane needs. Cars would require no modifications, nor would refineries, and there would be no energy penalty. MTBE is an oxygenate and these are already used in some countries, including the United States, either as octane boosters or as fuel extenders. Even the DOT admits that 'MTBE appears technically to be the most promising material, as it has few of the vices of methanol and does not lead to significant vehicle fuel system corrosion problems.'

LPG (liquid petroleum gas) is a mixture of propane and butane and compares favourably with petrol in price and is believed to be less damaging to the engine. It is simple to manufacture and of high octane. Cars need to be manufactured to run on it, although they can also run on petrol with a throw of a switch. The problem with LPG is availability. However, at least one local authority in Britain is already using it for its council fleet. This is practicable because local authority cars can all be fuelled from the same base and operate within a restricted area. If every local authority in the country, plus other big organisations with a fleet of cars operating within a restricted area, were to move to LPG, they would not only make considerable fuel economies, but more than balance any loss of energy caused by a move to lead-free petrol for the car population as a whole.

Diesel would be a completely alternative fuel. There would be no problem with supply. It is undoubtedly feasible and the long-term benefits would be a saving in energy consumption. For car owners a change to diesel engines would involve some initial expenditure balanced later by savings in running costs. Its widespread use would, however, have to be combined with effective control of other emissions so that diesel did not replace one environmental problem with another.

Finally, there are the filters. These, for reasons explained in chapter seven, I dismiss.

It is possible that, apart from the filters, there is a role for all the above options. What is clear is that lead-free petrol is a practical possibility, is already being achieved in other countries, is within the capability of both the British petroleum and car manufacturing industries, and that there are a variety of ways of proceeding towards it.

Opposition myths

Let us look now at some of the objections thrown up by the industries:

1 Price

If we proceed to low octane lead-free petrol, the price of petrol at the pump is not a problem. First, we know from the MORI poll that 80% of people are prepared to pay a few more pence per gallon for lead-free petrol.

Second, we know from BP that they can produce lead-free petrol for only about a penny a gallon more. Just what the additional cost of lead-free high octane is I cannot say, other than to report that the industry, whose claims have to be treated with considerable scepticism, claims that prices would increase substantially.

As, on balance, the low octane route is the most likely to be chosen, there clearly is no problem.

2 Performance

An Automobile Association survey of 14,000 drivers in Britain discovered that of the factors taken into account by car buyers, fuel economy was relatively low. Only one in five drivers named it as the most significant factor. In any case, we know that the Japanese have achieved exceptional fuel economy with lead-free petrol and a better performance in their own country with lead-free petrol than they can obtain in Britain with leaded petrol. The probability is, therefore, that this will not be an adverse factor at all.

3 Purchase price of car

If the high octane route is chosen, cars will require little modification and purchase prices will hardly be affected. If the low octane route is chosen, cars will require some adaptation. There will also be initial investment costs for the industry. At least one political party, Labour, has offered to consider assistance for the car manufacturers to meet these transition costs. It is important to emphasise that these transition costs would be once-and-for-all and that the sum mentioned by the industry of around £300 million is less than we were recently annually subsidising British Leyland alone. Ultimately, car prices would not be greatly affected – and not by as much as the cost of Government-imposed seat belts.

4   *Energy loss*
It is said that there will be a five per cent energy penalty if we move to lead-free petrol. When these calculations are made, the use of energy to make lead additives and transport them around the country, etc., are never included. In any event, the energy equation could easily be balanced out by my proposal of increased use of LPG for local fleets of vehicles and if incentives for use of MTBE and diesel were introduced for some cars.

5   *Benefit to overseas competitors*
It is said that while British car manufacturers are adapting to lead-free petrol, the Japanese would be able to flood the British market. This is a ludicrous scare story. Already the Japanese operate within voluntary undertakings about the number of cars they can export to Britain, and already British car manufacturers are calling for tighter controls on them to save the British car manufacturing industry. At the opening of the 1982 motor show, the President of the Society of Motor Manufacturers and Traders stated: 'I would like to point out that many countries currently outside the EEC, and which are exporting so energetically, have no qualms about protecting their own domestic markets. In no way do I advocate protectionism but I do advocate reciprocal trading arrangements.'
The introduction of lead-free petrol should make British car manufacturers more competitive. First, because this action would be taken for health reasons, the British authorities would have a unique opportunity to introduce import controls for a period of time on the grounds that 'as we have asked our car manufacturers to undertake a major programme of modification to protect the public health, we have to ask other countries to be understanding of the need for temporary protection.' This would probably be seen by overseas countries as a fair point provided it was not pushed too far, and would thus enable British car manufacturers to move to lead-free petrol without a sales penalty and in fact offer them the additional benefit of some protection in the domestic market place. Furthermore, British car manufacturers would then not have the additional costs of adapting some of their cars for Japanese, American, and

Australian markets, and would be well placed to prosper in the EEC market when Europe moves to lead-free petrol.

6 *British drivers would be in trouble when they travel to Europe because lead-free petrol is not available*
This is nonsense. A car manufactured to run on lead-free petrol will also run on leaded petrol.

There are, however, positive advantages in lead-free petrol for the car. Lead in petrol is not just the enemy of human beings; it is also the enemy of the car. On unleaded petrol, cars will run much longer between oil changes. Spark plugs last much longer. Exhaust systems do not rust so quickly. Eric Stork, who was responsible for the introduction of unleaded petrol on behalf of the EPA in America, states: 'On balance, there can be little doubt that our car owners are money ahead.'

Leaded petrol also obstructs any form of control of other pollutants. In March 1970 the technical advisory committee to the California State Air Resources Board presented a document on the removal of lead from petrol. It suggested that one of the ill effects of lead was that it increased other emissions from vehicles:

> Almost all possible emission control systems suffer some restraint from the presence of lead in fuel. . . . All published information on deposit formation and petrol engine combustion chambers is in accord that lead in gasoline contributes to the deposits which are built up. These deposits in turn increase the octane number requirement and progressively the amount of unburned hydrocarbon in the exhaust. Dupont and Ethyl Corporations (the two lead additive companies) report much lesser increments of increase in emissions than other organisations and differ in interpretation, but all studies thus far confirm these observations.
> One report indicated that there was as much as a 45% increase in hydrocarbon emission attributable to the deposit effect of lead alkyl in the petrol.
> A second effect of lead in fuel reported by the automobile companies is the inhibiting of exhaust system oxidation of hydrocarbons. This resulted in a small increase in hydrocarbon at the end of the exhaust pipe.
> Further factors through which lead in petrol is judged to influence present engine operation and emissions is fouling of spark plugs, and thus misfire, and intake valve deposits. Both of these can increase unburned hydrocarbons.
> The summation of the above effects results in the conclusion that reduction in concentration, or elimination of lead from petrol will reduce (other) emissions from the present population of motor vehicles.

A Ford Motor Car Company study in 1973 confirmed that . . .

> experiments have detected an immediate increase in hydrocarbon
> emissions on converting from non-leaded to leaded fuel. . . . Results
> showed a 35–50% increase in hydrocarbon levels with leaded fuel and
> essentially no increase with unleaded fuel.
> An examination of the engines involved in Ford's 1967–8 test indicates
> less piston-ring weight loss, less blow-by, less degradation of engine
> lubricant, and less deposits on spark plugs with operation on low lead
> compared to leaded fuel.

As far back as 1974, Dr. Vladimir Haensel, Vice-President,
Science and Technology, with Universal Oil Products Limited,
Illinois, was arguing about lead-free petrol that. . . .

> Driving tests show that the motorist may expect to derive a 3% increase
> in mileage from using it exclusively. Testimony by an official of the
> Standard Oil Company of Indiana before the House Sub-Committee
> on Public Health and Welfare in 1970 not only brought out the fact of
> the increased mileage but a significant saving in automobile mainten-
> ance – less corrosion of the exhaust system, freedom from combustion
> chamber deposits, longer-lived spark plugs and the like. All told,
> Indiana Standards representative reported a saving of 2–4 cents per
> gallon.

The New South Wales State Pollution Control Commission
published a leaflet in October 1980 entitled 'Lead-free petrol: How
you will benefit'. It stated:

> Lead-free petrol will reduce the cost of motoring in two ways: it will
> cut vehicle maintenance costs, and, by enabling the use of catalytic
> converters, it will lead to reduced fuel consumption. The removal of
> lead and lead scavengers from petrol will result in a longer life for
> engine and exhaust components and lubricating oil. Recent research
> indicates a saving in maintenance costs alone equivalent to 1 cent per
> litre of petrol.

Undoubtedly the most difficult decision for the CLEAR
campaign was whether to campaign for one route to lead-free petrol
or another. There is little question that the quickest way to lead-free
petrol would be the high octane route and on health grounds this
would have been our preference. We could not, however, press for
this for two reasons: first, on the evidence available we could not
prove that it could be done without incurring colossal costs. There
were those who told us it could, but they tended to be few and
unable to prove their case. On the other hand, the Japanese, the
Americans, and the Australians, had all investigated every possibility
and chosen the low octane route, and this was clearly the one

preferred by the car manufacturers and the petroleum industry if they were forced to act. Second, any responsible campaigner who genuinely wishes to achieve his objective will seek to find a balance between his ideal timescale and what can be sold to less-committed politicians and public.

It was proper that CLEAR should balance a sense of urgency for environmental protection with the political and economic realities. Therefore, we felt that it was best that we should concentrate on winning the decision to move towards lead-free petrol, and hope at that point that the industries could be forced to produce the relevant facts so that a well-informed decision could be taken on the quickest and most practical route to lead-free petrol.

As I have explained in chapter six, it was the need to carry the public with the campaign that led to our decision to call for a phasing out of lead in petrol so that existing cars could end their useful lives on leaded petrol if their owners wished. This too was a compromise. It recognised, however, that whatever our desires may be, the most likely choice of the authorities in Britain would be the same as the choice of other countries – low octane lead-free petrol.

If the low octane route is followed, then the following is possible:

(a) New cars in Britain could be manufactured to run on it.
(b) Lead-free petrol could be introduced in every petrol station alongside leaded petrol.
(c) The heavy tax on petrol could be loaded to the disadvantage of leaded petrol to encourage new car owners to use unleaded, and old car owners to use unleaded if possible, or to have their cars adapted.
(d) Tax incentives could be extended to LPG and diesel, and local authorities and other local car fleets encouraged to use LPG in particular to balance any overall energy loss.

At the same time as taking this decision Britain should campaign vigorously within the EEC to persuade other member countries to follow suit, and also introduce import controls for a limited period of time at present sales levels to protect our car manufacturing industry throughout the transition period. There will be complications and difficulties. But it can be done. It has been done in other countries, and it can be done in Britain.

First, however, the decision to eliminate lead from petrol has to be taken, for I have every confidence that if the industries are made to act, they will overcome the problems, and the penalties will be seen to be less than predicted. While they are campaigning to stop the introduction of unleaded petrol, the industries have an incentive to exaggerate the costs and difficulties; once they are made to act, they have an incentive to keep the costs to a minimum and overcome the difficulties efficiently and to their advantage (and thus, hopefully, the advantage of the consumer).

It really is a question of will, and that will has to be imposed upon them. From there on there is no major problem. As Dr. Needleman has written: 'Lead in the air is a product of man's activity and it can be controlled by man. Rarely do important biomedical problems offer themselves to such available remedy.'

PUTTING
PEOPLE FIRST ■

9.
A question of priorities

A simple test of the strength of the evidence incriminating lead in petrol as a health hazard is to ask this question:

> If lead had never been added to petrol, but this practice was now being proposed for the first time in the context of current knowledge of lead's health effects, would permission be given to proceed?

The answer must surely be 'no'.

This leads to another question:

> If the health evidence is such that we would not allow the practice to be *initiated* now, does it not also suggest that even now it should be stopped?

Unfortunately, at this stage factors other than health enter the decision-making process. Before lead was added to petrol, unleaded petrol was the status quo. Now the opposite is the case. And, as one academic, D.G.Collingridge has pointed out, '*the entrenchment of technology means that in the debate about changes, the status quo has an unfair advantage*'.

In an article in 1979 he described what happens when technology, such as that of leaded petrol, becomes entrenched.

Entrenchment means that the timing of change is fixed. 'In reviewing the problem of reducing lead additives in petrol, one cannot but be struck by the impression that the time of change is determined more by the technology itself than by human intervention. . . . In the case of a possible environmental hazard like lead, these unavoidable delays may mean that the population is subjected to considerable harm.' Entrenchment means that change is hotly debated. 'Why is the reduction of lead additive in petrol so contentious an issue? Surely because such a reduction will be very expensive, but it will be expensive and also protracted because of the way in which lead additive technology has become entrenched. Were it not for this entrenchment, the reduction of lead levels would be so straightforward an issue that debate on the scale which we see today would be quite superfluous.'

He continues: 'In a world so much tidier than the real one, the scientific task of determining whether or not lead from petrol is harmful would be separated from the political one of deciding how much money to spend on remedying the situation. In our more chaotic world, however, these two aspects of the problem become conflated. Because the reduction of lead-levels in petrol will be costly and protracted, *the scientific case against lead has to be made very much stronger before being accepted than it would otherwise be.*'

Finally, he points out that entrenchment means that 'fixes' are strongly favoured. 'If some way could be found of alleviating the problem which gives rise to the call for change in an entrenched technology without actually making the change, it is obviously going to be received very favourably.' Thus the Whitehall preference for a compromise lead level, or for a filter.

Undoubtedly, Collingridge was correct in identifying the environmentalists' problem with lead in petrol as a confrontation with entrenched technology. What, then is the first lesson to be learned from the lead in petrol controversy? It is that there should be a far greater burden of proof on industry to prove that any new practices are safe *before* they are introduced. In this way, the dangers of entrenchment can be averted.

A feature of the lead in petrol issue is that the burden of proof has been placed on we, the citizens, to demonstrate that lead in petrol is dangerous; the industries have not been called upon to demonstrate that it is safe. Indeed, as I have shown, both the car manufacturing and the petroleum industries have washed their hands of any responsibility on the health issue. 'We are not qualified to judge', they say. This simply won't do. Their refusal to participate in the health debate, and the failure of the British political system to force them to argue that their product is safe, is evidence that in many respects our governmental system is biased towards organisational interests rather than those of the individual.

Another lesson from the lead in petrol controversy is that Britain has not developed an effective environmental defence mechanism. This is reflected in the way the decision on lead in petrol is shared by a variety of Ministries. The DOE are responsible (some would say irresponsible) for environmental protection. The DHSS is responsible for health. The Education Ministry is concerned where there is evidence of damage to children's ability to learn. The Energy Ministry is involved because of the energy implications, and the Transport Ministry for obvious reasons. The Exchequer is involved because of the financial implications, and even the Foreign Office can enter into the debate because of the EEC implications. In the case of lead in petrol, it is known that the Ministries most responsible for the environmental and health issues, the DOE and the DHSS, actually recommended the fixing of a date for lead-free petrol in the pre-May 1981 days and were over-ruled by the others. They simply did not have the political strength, or the strength of character, to stand and fight and were easily out-gunned in Whitehall. A document circulated within the Energy Ministry in 1980 and leaked to CLEAR stated:

> Other Departments have continued to argue that lead in petrol should bear the full brunt of the Government's response to Lawther. The Department of Transport, the DOE, and the DHSS lead in proposing immediate action to reduce the lead limit to 0.15 grams per litre with further commitment to lead-free petrol.

(Incidentally, Whitehall's apathy on lead pollution was revealed by another paragraph in this memo. It said: 'The action on the other sources of lead exposure which the responsible Departments are prepared to disclose is limited to publicising the dangers, rather than eliminating the problem. Other Departments are not prepared to incur the cost of remedial action.')

It is significant that both DOE and DHSS spokesmen repeatedly talk about the economic implications of taking lead out of petrol. These should not be their priorities. What chance have environmental and public health causes if the Ministries responsible for them so easily adopt the language and priorities of the Treasury.

The US Environmental Protection Agency may not be perfect, but there is an overwhelming case for taking environmental and health protection responsibilities out of the conventional Whitehall machine and placing them in the hands of an agency with genuine independence and a genuine concern for the health of the citizen.

I do not reach this judgement on the lead issue alone. One can point to many other instances of the failure of the system. One is well described by Judith Cook and Chris Kaufman in their history of the 2,4,5-T story. They report:

> One of the most damaging indictments of 2,4,5-T came in 1980 from the US Environmental Protection Agency. It has accumulated reams of evidence, waded through mountains of cases, records and research. Its conclusions stated: 'The quality, quantity and variety of data demonstrating that the continued use of 2,4,5-T contaminated with dioxin presents risks to human health is unprecedented and overwhelming'. Yet in Britain the Government refuses to ban its use. You can buy it from your local garden shop to use in your garden. . . . In December 1978 the EEC issued a Directive banning 67 pesticide products as being too dangerous to use. All had been approved by the various British agencies which are supposed to clear such substances. . . . For those who have been involved in the debate it has often proved difficult to distinguish between the voices of the spokesmen for the agro-chemicals industry and those of the Ministry of Agriculture.

Exchange the word 'lead' for '2,4,5-T' and one could be making exactly the same points in almost exactly the same words. *The Observer* reported in November 1982 that the EEC wanted to introduce new restrictions on 2,4,5-T. A Commission spokesman was quoted as saying 'Clearly this stuff is absolutely lethal'. However, *The Observer* reported, the British were strongly contesting the Commission's conclusions and opposing European laws on the use of pesticides. As there was no European legislation on pesticide use, the Commission was likely to be forced to back down when Britain refused to accept even minor restrictions.

I have already referred more than once to asbestos. As Cook and Kaufman comment:

> Gravestones cover the victims of asbestos. The first case of asbestosis was diagnosed in 1906. By the 1930s our own Health and Safety Inspectorate had named asbestos as a carcinogen and some American companies were settling claims out of court. Yet in 1976 the British asbestos industry increased its publicity budget from £55,000 to £500,000 and embarked on a national public relations campaign, some of the advertisements later having to be withdrawn. Official estimates in America put the potential deaths from asbestos exposure among workers at 2 million. In Britain it is estimated at 500,000.

Yet only in 1982 after a major television programme had shown the damage being done to human beings by asbestos did the Government even take tentative steps towards greater protection.

The extent that major industries can dictate to democratically-elected Governments was illustrated by the behaviour of the tobacco industry in 1982. The Government decided to ask the tobacco industry to publish tougher health warnings on cigarette packets stating: 'Smoking causes bronchitis, lung cancer and heart disease'. The tobacco industry refused. The Health Minister, Kenneth Clarke (yes, he who shares responsibility for the continuation of lead pollution in Britain), was quoted in *The Guardian* as saying that 'a voluntary agreement was the best we could achieve in a democracy'. Why should this be so? Government has no difficulty in imposing its will on ordinary citizens. Why is it impossible to do so when dealing with big industries?

Further, the Government insisted on a contribution of £11 million to health research from the tobacco industry, but, reported *The Guardian*, while the money would be concentrated on health promotion to encourage young people to be more responsive to health problems and to investigate environmental and social factors governing health care, 'researchers accepting the cash will be banned, at the industry's insistence, from investigating the use and effects of tobacco'.

The British Medical Association was quoted as condemning the terms of reference for the research fund:

> The limitation on the activities of the Trust is disgraceful. Medical evidence has continued to show that smoking is responsible for major and extensive areas of disease in addition to lung cancer . . . the tobacco industry should not be allowed to attempt to buy off its responsibilities in this way.

This is a classic case of the weakness of Whitehall and Westminster in the face of the industrial lobby. The system isn't working, and it isn't working because environmental and public health protection still does not warrant sufficient priority in Britain, and because Whitehall is over-influenced by industry behind the scenes. There is a huge bias within the British bureaucracy towards the status quo, and an arrogance that allows them to believe that they know best and that they can trample over the evidence that is contrary to their views. Power in Whitehall is, above all, vested in the Treasury and its social conscience is nil.

In his summing up of the US Court of Appeal's case on lead in petrol in 1976, Circuit Judge, J. Skelly writes:

> Man's ability to alter his environment has developed far more rapidly than his ability to foresee with certainty the effects of his alterations. It is only recently that we have begun to appreciate the danger posed by

unregulated modification of the world around us, and have created watchdog agencies whose task it is to warn us, and protect us, when technological 'advances' present dangers unappreciated – or unrevealed – by their supporters. Such agencies, unequipped with crystal balls and unable to read the future, are nonetheless charged with evaluating the effects of unprecedented environmental modifications, often made on a massive scale. Necessarily, they must deal with predictions and uncertainty, with developing evidence, with conflicting evidence and sometimes, with little or no evidence at all.

The fact is that we in Britain do not have an adequate 'watchdog agency' and the time has come to demand one. The lead in petrol controversy has demonstrated that we cannot look to those responsible for public health to objectively weigh the evidence and to have an in-built prejudice towards environmental and health protection. On the contrary, one of the most disturbing aspects of the whole controversy has been the way civil servants, having made a disastrous decision, were prepared to wage war to defend it, irrespective of the accumulating evidence. They were prepared to use the power of the Governmental propaganda machine to mislead public opinion, and the sloth or stupidity of their Ministers to broadcast unquestioningly the mis-information placed before them.

It is not enough, however, to blame the authorities, because at least to some extent, they represent the priorities of society as a whole. The British, and indeed Europe as a whole, have to be alerted to the negative side of the technological changes that are taking place. The ability of huge multi-national industries to pollute the air we breathe, the water we drink, and the food we eat, and not only undermine our own health, but threaten even more the health of generations to come, has become colossal. Too often environmentalists are cast as 'idealists', as if it is over-idealistic, or radical, to want to protect the health of one's children; too often environmental issues are seen as fringe issues, when in fact they are central to man's health and survival. It is incumbent upon each of us to understand these matters and to make clear our priorities. We must insist that people come first.

When it comes to the subject of this book, lead in petrol, I believe any reasonable, open-minded person would accept that there *is* overwhelming evidence that lead at low levels of exposure *does* represent a danger to children, that lead in petrol *is* an unacceptable pollutant, and that its elimination *is* practicable. Our human priorities should complete the story.

Key publications

Key Publications

1 Lead Versus Health: Low Level Lead Exposure and Its Effect on Human Beings – Proceedings of the CLEAR International Symposium held in London, May 10–12, 1982 M. Rutter & R. Russel Jones (eds) (Wiley & Sons) (1983)

2 Low Level Lead Exposure: The Clinical Implications of Current Research, Raven Press (1980) H. L. Needleman (ed).

3 Lead in the Human Environment: US National Academy of Science, Washington DC, USA (1980)

4 Air Quality Criteria for Lead: Office of Research and Development, US Environmental Protection Agency, Washington DC, USA (1977)

5 Lead and Health: Department of Health and Social Security – The Report of a DHSS Working Party on Lead in the Environment (1980) HMSO (Chairman: Professor Patrick Lawther)

6 Lead or Health: A Review of Contemporary Lead Pollution and a Commentary on the DHSS Report 'Lead and Health' prepared for the Conservation Society by D. Bryce-Smith and R. Stephens (1981). (Published by the Conservation Society, 68 Dora Road, London SW19)

7 Effects of Lead in the Canadian Environment: 1978 Executive Report by J. F. Jaworski, National Research Council, Canada

Papers

1 H. L. Needleman et al – Deficits in Psychologic and Classroom Performance of Children With Elevated Dentine Lead Levels.

Reprinted from the New England Journal of Medicine Vol. 300, pp. 689–695, March 29, 1979

2   I. H. Billick, A. S. Curran, D. R. Shier – Relation of Pediatric Blood Lead Levels to Lead in Gasoline. In: Environmental Health Perspectives, Vol. 34, pp. 213–217, 1980

3   G. Winneke – Neurobehavioural and Neuropsychological Effects of Lead. Paper presented at CLEAR International Symposium, May 10–12, 1982. In: 'Lead Versus Health' edited by M. Rutter and R. Russell Jones

4   M. Rutter – Raised Lead Levels and Impaired Cognitive/ Behavioural Functioning: A Review of the Evidence. Supplement to: Developmental Medicine and Child Neurology Vol. 22, No. 1 (Publication date, March 1, 1980)

5   R. Lansdown, W. Yule, M. Urbanowicz, I. Millar – Relationships Between Blood-Lead, Intelligence, Attainment and Behaviour in School Children: Overview of a Pilot Study. Paper presented at CLEAR International Symposium, London, May 10–12, 1982. In: 'Lead Versus Health' edited by M. Rutter and R. Russell Jones

6   J. Lee Annest et al – Blood-Lead Levels for Persons 6 Months– 74 Years of Age: United States 1976–80 (NHANES 11 survey). From: Vital and Health Statistics of the National Center for Health Statistics, USA, No. 79, May 12, 1982

7   EEC Commission – Isotopic Lead Experiment: Status Report prepared by S. Facchette & F. Geiss, Joint Research Centre, Ispra, Italy, July 1982

8   US Federal Register – Part V: Environmental Protection Agency Regulation of Fuels and Fuel Additives. August 27, 1982

Index